YOGA

YOUR HOME PRACTICE COMPANION

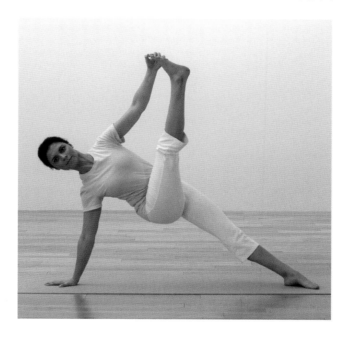

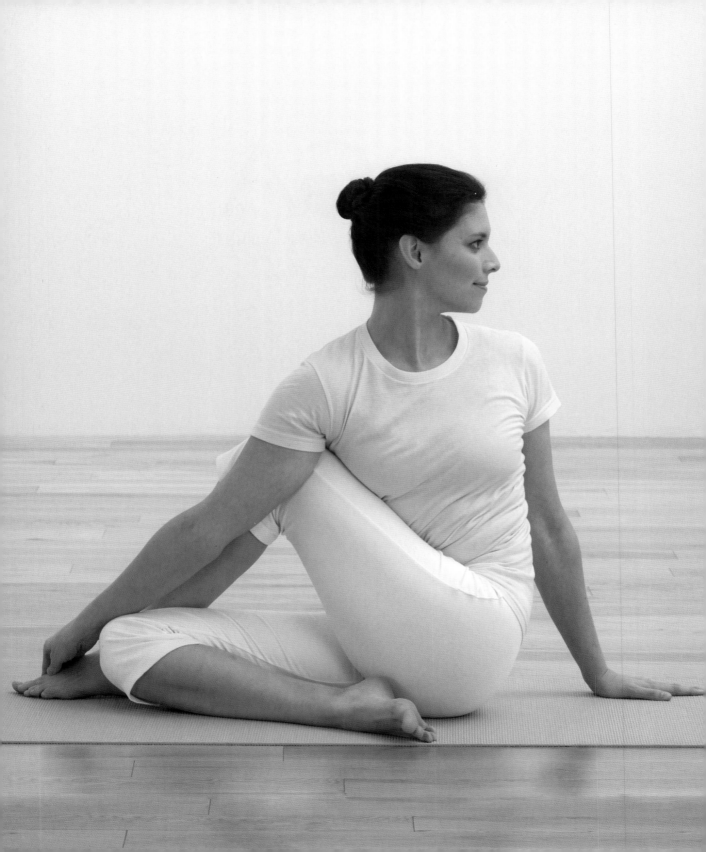

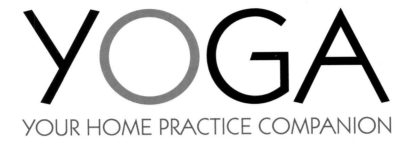

YOGA

YOUR HOME PRACTICE COMPANION

Sivananda Yoga Vedanta Centre

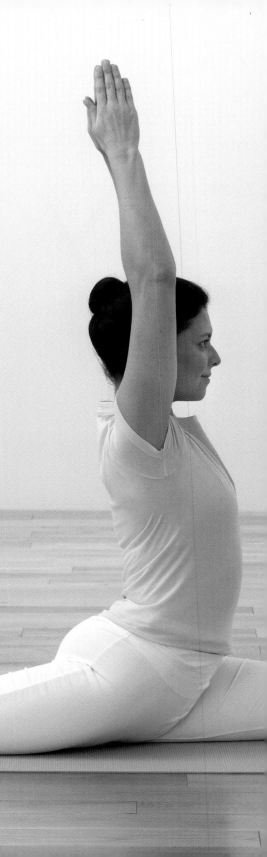

London, New York, Melbourne, Munich, and Delhi

For H.H. Sri Swami Vishnudevananda

Contributors from the Sivananda Yoga Vedanta Centre
Swami Durgananda
Swami Kailasananda
Swami Sivasananda

Project Editor Hilary Mandleberg
Senior Editor Jennifer Latham
Senior Art Editor Susan Downing
Designers Danaya Bunnag, Caroline de Souza,
   Mandy Earey, Anne Fisher, Helen McTeer
Managing Editor Dawn Henderson
Managing Art Editor Christine Keilty
Senior Jacket Creative Nicola Powling
Art Director Peter Luff
Publisher Mary-Clare Jerram
DTP Designer Sonia Charbonnier
Senior Production Controller Alice Holloway
Senior Production Editor Ben Marcus

Illustrations Peter Bull Arts Studio

First published in Great Britain in 2010
by Dorling Kindersley Limited
80 Strand, London WC2R 0RL

Penguin Group (UK)

Health warning
All participants in fitness activities must assume the
responsibility for their own actions and safety. If you have
any health problems or medical conditions, consult with
your physician before undertaking any of the activities set
out in this book. The information contained in this book
cannot replace sound judgement and good decision
making, which can help reduce risk of injury.

A CIP catalogue record for this book is
available from the British Library

ISBN 978-1-4053-4918-5

Printed and bound in China by South China Co. Ltd

Discover more at **www.dk.com**

Sivananda Yoga Vedanta Centre
www.sivananda.org

Contents

Introduction 6

An Ancient Guide to Healthy Living • What is Yoga? • The Yogic Path to Well-being • Hatha Yoga Pradipika

The Benefits of Yoga 16

Boosting Self-Healing • Muscles and Movement • Aligning the Posture • The Breath of Life • Supporting the Nervous System • Yoga and the Endocrine System • Yoga and Relaxation • One Pose, Many Benefits

Proper Exercise 42

What is Proper Exercise? • Initial Relaxation • Eye and Neck Exercises • Sun Salutation • Single Leg Lifts • Double Leg Lifts • Headstand • Shoulderstand • Plough • Fish • Forward Bend • Cobra • Locust • Bow • Half Spinal Twist • Crow • Peacock • Standing Forward Bend • Triangle • Beginner Programmes • Intermediate Programmes • Advanced Programmes

Proper Breathing 176

Pranayama • Preparatory Exercises • Alternate Nostril Breathing • Kapala Bhati

Proper Relaxation 186

Relaxation Between Asanas • Final Relaxation • Complete Yogic Relaxation

Positive Thinking and Meditation 196

Why Meditate? • The Art of Concentration • Practising Meditation • Managing Stress • The Law of Karma

Proper Diet 208

Yoga and Vegetarianism • You are What You Eat • Common Concerns About the Yogic Diet • The Transition Towards a Yogic Diet • Cooking Techniques • A Week's Menu Plan • Breakfast • Lunch • Salads and Dressings • Vegetables and Condiments • Dinner • Breads • Sweet Treats and Desserts • Snacks and Beverages

Resources 250

Index 252

Acknowledgments 256

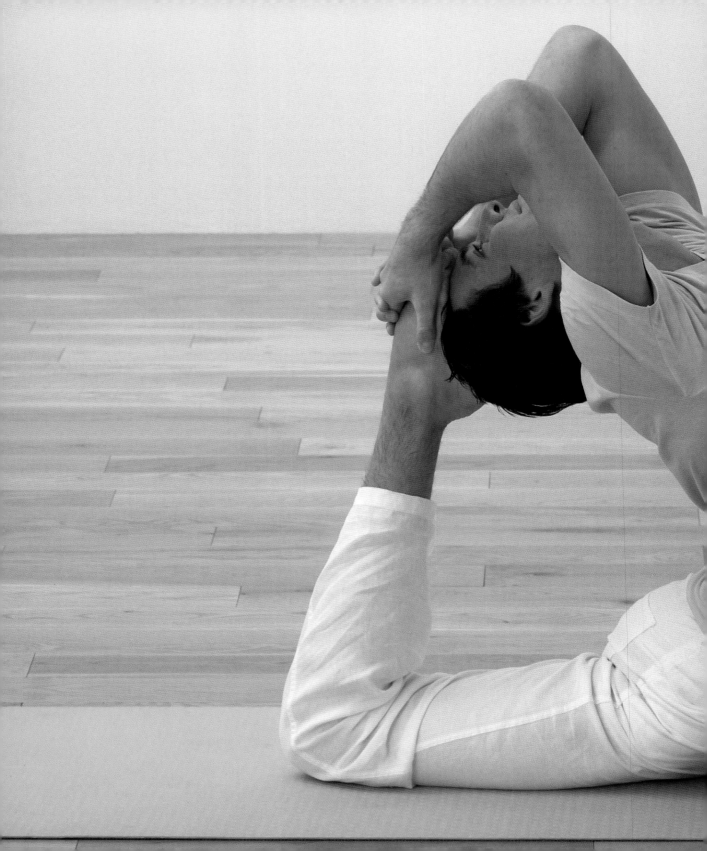

Introduction

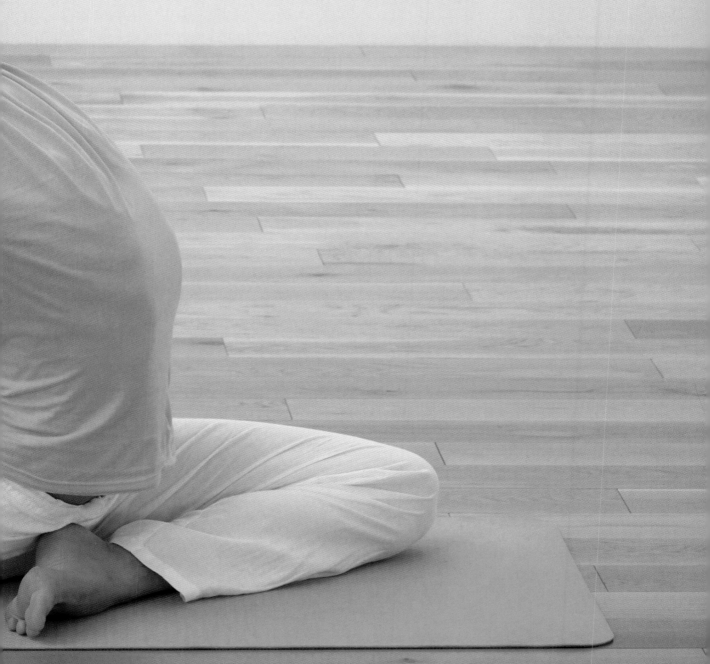

An ancient guide to healthy living

Yoga is a centuries-old guide to healthy living developed by ancient Indian sages. With its unique blend of physical exercises, psychological insight, and philosophy, it can help you to bring your body, mind, and spirit into better balance. Yoga takes a holistic approach to life, enabling you to experience complete equilibrium inside and out.

Yoga for everyone

For centuries, yoga was open only to people who were ready to search for a teacher in India, and traditionally it only appealed to those willing to forego the life of a "householder", renouncing the world and living in seclusion. H.H. Swami Sivananda (1887–1963) and Swami Vishnudevananda (1927–1993) were among the first of the Indian yoga masters to make yoga accessible to anyone, no matter their background, age, or status, or where in the world they lived. In doing so, they helped to bring yoga to the West.

Swami Sivananda

Sri Swami Sivananda was a practising doctor who was eager to do all he could to relieve human misery. In a search to ease his patients' physical and mental discomfort, he decided to look within himself. He began his quest by becoming a swami – a wandering monk – and after long years of secluded practice in the Himalayas, he attained mastery in yoga and meditation. Swami Sivananda went on to found the Divine Life Society in Rishikesh, in the Himalayas. Here, he trained students from many countries and various religions in a synthesis of the key paths of yoga, encompassing Hatha and Raja Yoga, Karma Yoga, Bhakti Yoga, and Jnana Yoga (see pp10–11). He also wrote more than 200 books in English explaining the most complex aspects of yoga in simple, practical terms.

Swami Vishnudevananda and the West

Swami Vishnudevananda was a close disciple of Swami Sivananda and an adept in the practice of Hatha and Raja Yoga (see p10). In 1957, Swami Sivananda commanded him to, "Go to the West, people are waiting".

"Yoga is a science perfected by the ancient seers of India, not of India merely, but of humanity as a whole. It is an exact science. It is a perfect, practical system of self-culture."
Swami Sivananda

With no means of support other than his faith and a remarkable energy, Swami Vishnudevananda travelled to North America, Europe, and many other parts of the world, where he became a pioneer in yoga, spreading the teachings of his master.

Swami Vishnudevananda founded the International Sivananda Yoga Vedanta Centres at the heart of many of the world's capital cities. Here, people are able to learn yoga as they go about their daily lives. Swami Vishnudevananda also established several ashrams (yoga retreats) in beautiful natural settings around the globe, from the forested mountains of Canada to Paradise Island in the Bahamas. He promoted yoga vacation programmes, which offer people an opportunity to learn the yogic disciplines while enjoying a healthy and relaxing holiday.

After experiencing a vision during meditation, Swami Vishnudevananda felt compelled to start up a campaign for world peace, which became known as T.W.O., True World Order. It adopted the mottos, "United we live – divided we perish" and "Cross man-made borders with flowers and love, not with bombs and guns". Swami Vishnudevananda learnt how to pilot a small plane and flew over many of the world's conflict zones, showering them with flowers and leaflets promoting the universal love taught by all the world's great religions. Two memorable flights took him over the Suez canal during the Sinai War in 1971 and over the Berlin Wall from West Germany to East Germany in 1983.

Teacher training

As part of his vision of yoga for world peace, Swami Vishnudevananda taught the first yoga teachers' training course in the West, in 1969. As well as offering a broad study of yoga philosophy, psychology, and teaching techniques, the four-week residential programme focused on an intense personal practice of yoga and meditation. It is even more popular today than during Swami Vishnudevananda's lifetime. Since the training course was founded, more than 25,000 graduates from all walks of life and every continent have taken the yoga teachings of Swami Vishnudevananda and Swami Sivananda back into their own communities.

The defining feature of this approach to yoga is its simplicity: regardless of age, physique, and walk of life, anyone can benefit from this step-by-step guide to asana (exercise), pranayama (breathing), relaxation, diet, positive thinking, and meditation. These key teachings are outlined in the chapters of this book to help you, too, to experience this ancient way of bringing balance into every aspect of your life.

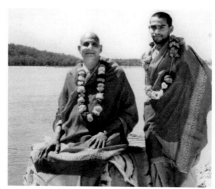

A JOURNEY BEGINS
Shortly before his departure to the West, Swami Vishnudevananda stands beside his master, Swami Sivananda.

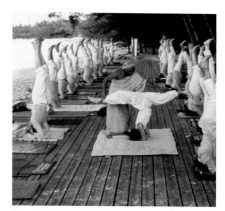

TRAINING THE TEACHERS
An asana class during a teachers' training course in Nassau, The Bahamas. Swami Vishnudevananda works with a student.

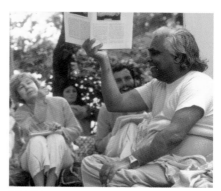

PIONEERING WORK
Swami Vishnudevananda was one of the first Indian master yogis to spread the teaching of yoga across the western world.

What is yoga?

Traditionally, there are four paths of yoga. Although each of them is a complete discipline in itself, it is best not to follow one path only. Combining the four practices helps the emotional, intellectual, and physical aspects of your life to develop in harmony.

The four paths of yoga

Of the four yogic paths, in the West only one is generally well-known and widely practised – the physical and mind-focusing path of Hatha and Raja Yoga, which includes postures and breathing exercises.

HATHA AND RAJA YOGA This is the yogic path of body and mind control. It is best known for its practical aspects, particularly its asanas (postures) and pranayama (breathing exercises). This path teaches ways of controlling the body and mind, including silent meditation, and its practices gradually transform the energy of the body and mind into spiritual energy. This path suits people who are looking for inner and outer transformation.

KARMA YOGA This is the yogic path of action and you practise it when you act selflessly, without thinking about success or reward. This path is valued for purifying the heart and reducing the influence of the ego on your words, actions, and interaction with others. Practising Karma Yoga is the best way to prepare yourself for silent meditation (see pp202–204). It suits people with an active, outgoing temperament.

BHAKTI YOGA This is the yogic path of devotion. It involves prayer, worship, and ritual, including chanting and singing devotional songs, and those who practise it eventually come to experience God as the embodiment of love. This yogic path has great appeal for people who are emotional by nature.

JNANA YOGA This is the yogic path of wisdom or knowledge, and it involves studying the philosophy of Vedanta – one of the six classical Indian philosophies. It teaches ways to examine the self and analyse human nature. The goal of this form of yoga is to recognize the Supreme Self in yourself and in all beings. This path is best suited to intellectual people, and is considered by many to be the most challenging path.

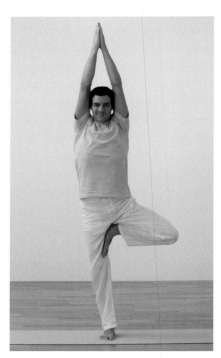

HATHA AND RAJA YOGA IN ACTION
This path includes the practice of asanas. Each asana requires a specific balance of posture, breathing, and relaxation.

The eight steps of Hatha and Raja Yoga

This path was codified by the ancient sage Patanjali in his *Yoga Sutras* as an eight-step training system for body and mind, which he called Ashtanga Yoga (in Sanskrit, *ashta* is "eight" and *anga* "division" or "limb"). The steps purify body and mind until enlightenment occurs.

1 YAMA Sets out the actions from which yogis should restrain. It advocates living a life of non-violence and truthfulness, sublimating sexual energy, not stealing, and not accepting gifts or bribes.

2 NIYAMA Details the actions a yogi should do. It advocates external and internal cleanliness, contentment, self-discipline, study of spiritual literature, and devotion to God. Together, the yamas and niyamas form a highly moral code of ethical conduct. Following them makes the mind more positive and purifies it, ready for deep meditation.

3 ASANA The third step relates to posture. The 12 basic asanas and their variations prepare the body for the meditative poses that are used in steps 6, 7 and 8 (see below).

4 PRANAYAMA The fourth step concerns control of *prana* or life energy. This is achieved by doing deep-breathing exercises, which include practising breath retention (see pp182–5).

5 PRATYAHARA Steps 3 and 4 project the practitioner into a world of intense inner perception. Step 5 teaches how to stabilize this withdrawal of the senses as a preparation to concentration.

6 DHARANA In this step, concentration, the mind is fixed on an imaginary or real object to the exclusion of other thoughts. This is the key practice in all yoga meditation techniques (see pp200–204).

7 DHYANA Step 6 leads to step 7, meditation. This uninterrupted flow of thought waves has been compared to oil flowing in an unbroken, stream from one container to another.

8 SAMADHI The final step happens effortlessly as, during meditation, the mind is absorbed into Absolute Consciousness, beyond all the usual states of waking, dreaming, and deep sleep (p198).

"You can have calmness of mind at all times by the practice of yoga. You can have restful sleep. You can have increased energy, vigour, vitality, longevity, and a high standard of health. You can turn out efficient work within a short space of time. You can have success in every walk of life."

Swami Sivananda

The yogic path to well-being

Swami Vishnudevananda taught five easy principles of yoga, all of which are explained in different chapters in this book. They bring together the often-complex philosophies and teachings of India's ancient yogis in a form that is easy to understand and simple to adapt to everyday life, wherever you live in the world.

The five principles of yoga

If you follow these five easy principles, said Swami Vishnudevananda, you will improve your physical and mental health and deepen your connection with the spiritual aspects of life.

Proper exercise

Asanas (see pp42–169) rejuvenate the whole body. They work primarily on the spine and central nervous system. The spine gains in strength and flexibility, and circulation is stimulated, bringing nutrients and oxygen to all the cells of the body. Asanas increase motion in the joints and flexibility in muscles, tendons, and ligaments. They massage internal organs, boosting their function.

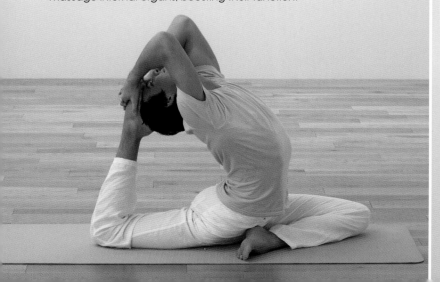

Proper breathing

Pranayama (see pp176–85) stimulates the energy reserves of the solar plexus, revitalizing body and mind. Regulating the breath helps to store prana, laying down reserves of strength and vitality. Deep, conscious breathing helps to conquer depression and stress, and controlling prana – by controlling the breath – can relieve symptoms of illness in a similar way to acupuncture.

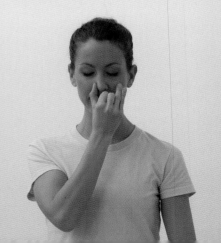

Proper relaxation

Deep relaxation (see pp186–95) works on three levels – physical, mental, and spiritual – and is the most natural way to re-energize body and mind. Regular relaxation acts like a car's cooling system, keeping the engine from over-heating and ensuring the vehicle functions efficiently. During the deep relaxation at the end of a yoga session, the body uses only enough prana to maintain vital metabolic activities. The rest of the energy gained during practice is stored.

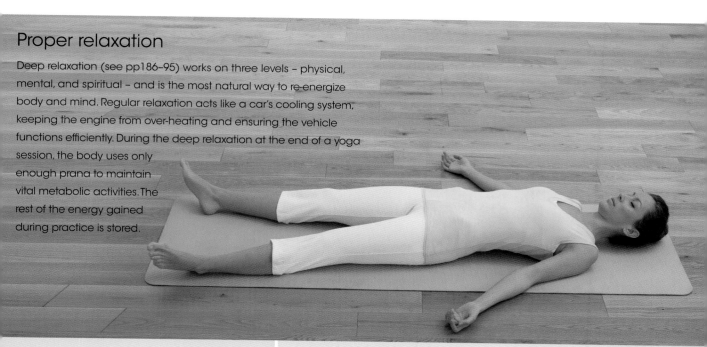

Proper diet

The yogic attitude to food (see pp208–49) is eat to live, not live to eat. Yogis choose foods with a positive effect on body and mind, and least negative effects on the environment and other creatures. A lacto-vegetarian diet is recommended – grains, pulses, fruits and vegetables, nuts, seeds, and dairy products – including plenty of plants. Fresh and unrefined foods are thought best, prepared simply, to preserve maximum nutrients.

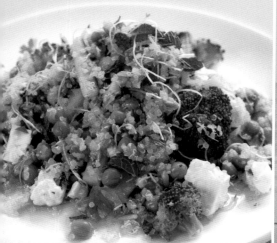

Positive thinking and meditation

Positive thinking and meditation (see pp196–207) are the yogic keys to peace of mind. Meditation techniques calm the mind and enhance focus. Regular meditation promotes physical and spiritual, as well as mental, well-being. Before meditation, yoga practitioners clear the mind of negative thoughts and feelings, using concentration and positive-thinking exercises.

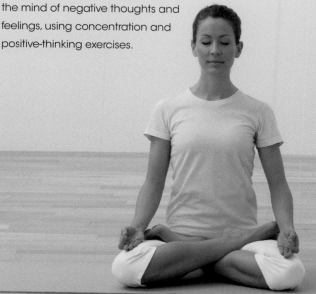

The Hatha Yoga Pradipika

The oldest surviving of the texts on Hatha Yoga, the *Hatha Yoga Pradipika* is said to have been written down by Swatmarama Yogi in the 15th century, although it is derived from earlier sources. Despite being more than five centuries old, the advice given in this manual on postures, breathing exercises, and the philosophy of yoga is still relevant today, whether you are a beginner or a more experienced practitioner.

Selected extracts

These six extracts from the *Hatha Yoga Pradipika* – which translates as "Light on Hatha Yoga" – have been selected to inspire your practice. Commentaries suggest how to apply them to deepen your experience of yoga.

Swatmarama Yogi, having saluted his own teacher, gives out the Hatha Vidya [knowledge] solely for the attainment of Raja Yoga. 12

This passage stresses the importance of thinking of your practice as a way of controlling the mind – this is the path of Hatha and Raja Yoga (see p10). Many in the West regard asanas as a form of physical exercise only, but practising them in this way is not to be recommended. It is impossible to master the mind without first controlling its physical counter-part, the body. This is what we seek to do when practising postures. The connection between body and mind is one of the most fascinating aspects of yoga.

Asanas make one firm, free from disease, and light of limb. 117

This explains how beneficial *asana* practice is. The "firmness" is seen in many ways, including improved alignment, increased resistance to heat and cold, hunger and thirst, and greater capacity for self-healing. Lightness of limb does not mean only physical weight (although asana practice does help maintain an ideal weight), but the ability of asanas to raise the vibratory level of the body's energy. This is seen in movement: if someone with a large frame practises asanas, a new lightness appears in their movements.

Moderate diet is defined to mean taking pleasant and sweet food, leaving one-fourth of the stomach free, and offering the act up to Siva. I 58

Here, we are told that a moderate, nutritious, and light diet is key to success in yoga. Easily digested, fresh vegetarian foods, simply cooked, are thought to be a good source of prana, or life force. Swami Sivananda advised that the way to be always happy is always to feel a little hungry.

When the breath wanders, i.e., is irregular, the mind is also unsteady, but when the breath is still, so is the mind, and the yogi lives long. So one should restrain the breath. II 2

Breath control is central to yoga: the term *Hatha* means "union of the sun (*Ha*) and the moon (*Tha*)", where sun and moon refer to inhalation and exhalation respectively. Both asanas and pranayama provide excellent training for the breath, which increases vital energy, fine-tunes the nervous system, and eventually leads to control of the mind.

He should gradually inhale the breath and as gradually exhale it. He should also restrain it gradually. II 18

This highlights the real hallmark of an accomplished practitioner of yoga. Strength and flexibility in postures are not by themselves a sign of progress. A smooth, rhythmical, balanced breath is. But never make any violent effort to control the breath in your yoga practice; this strains the nervous system.

The Yogi succeeds by cheerfulness, perseverance, courage, true knowledge, firm belief in the words of the guru, and by abandoning bad company. I 16

Making yoga practice your own by having the right "knowledge" and "firm belief" (of the five principles, see pp12–13) opens the door to new friendships with like-minded people. The purpose of yoga is to shift your life force from a dormant or static state to a dynamic state. This requires perseverance, self-discipline, and courage.

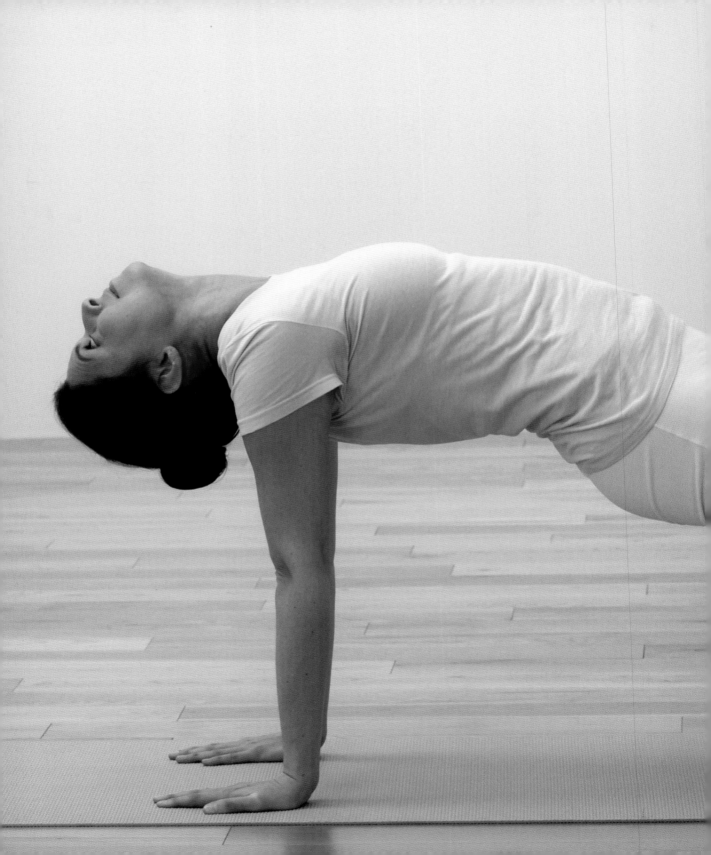

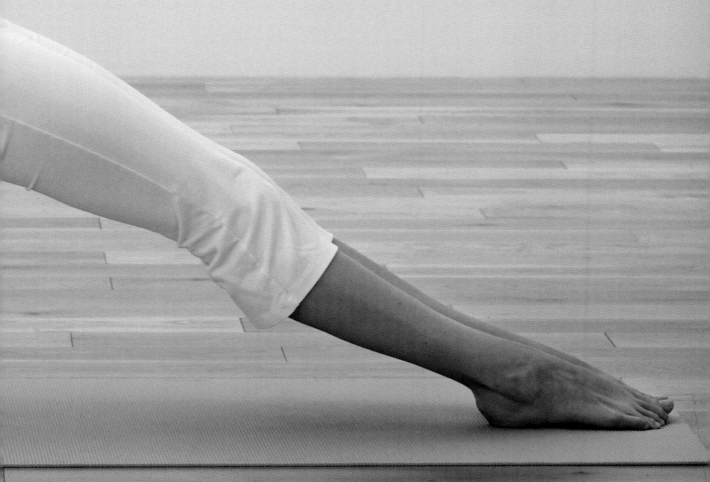

The Benefits
of Yoga

Boosting self-healing

The human body is superbly intelligent. It manages to maintain an intricate physiological balance day and night, through every stage of life. Practising yoga helps the body to maintain this complex balance, which boosts your capacity for self-healing.

The study of physiology shows that the nervous and the endocrine systems (see pp34–7) ensure that the body's other major systems, such as the digestive and respiratory systems, all cooperate in an "intelligent" way. The result is "homeostasis", derived from Greek and meaning "remaining the same". When homeostasis is achieved, there is perfect balance between the various body functions and, as long as the body has a regular supply of food and water and is not over-taxed physically, it tends naturally towards self-healing. Ancient yogis described a different but equally complex system of homeostasis in the body, based on a finely tuned balance of the five elements: earth, water, fire, air, and "ether" or space (see right). When these elements are in equilibrium, again body and mind tend towards self-healing.

The causes of disease

Why, then, does the body succumb to illness, even in parts of the world where there is no scarcity of food or water and where people do not have to do hard physical labour? According to yoga, the chief cause of disease lies in difficult emotions, such as anxiety, desire, anger, hatred, and jealousy. These disturb the body's natural balance and can lead to unhealthy lifestyle choices, from overeating to smoking. These, in turn, are factors in many diseases common in modern societies, from heart disease to diabetes.

Balancing the emotions

Practising positive thinking and meditation (see pp196–207) makes it less likely that you will be affected by negative emotions and the lifestyle choices they lead to. But it is easier to meditate and think positively if you first pay attention to the body, practising yoga asanas, or postures (see pp42–169), pranayama, or breathing exercises (see pp176–85), and relaxation (see pp186–95). You can also support your health by eating well (see pp208–49).

All these elements come together in yoga. In fact, the Sanskrit word *yoga* means "union". Practising yoga helps the body to find its natural balance and teaches the mind to be a responsible and intelligent driver of the body.

The five elements

Traditional yogic texts describe the body as a "food sheath" (*anayamaya kosha*), made up of five elements. We maintain health by constantly adjusting the body to bring it into harmony with these five elements.

Earth Bones, muscles, and skin contain this element. Asanas move the earth element in all possible directions.

Water Mainly relates to blood. Asanas improve circulation, balance blood pressure, and strengthen the heart.

Fire Seen in the 36–39°C (97–102°F) range of internal temperatures that the body can survive. Practising yoga adapts the body to climatic change.

Air Yoga improves the circulation of air in the body. Breathing exercises increase the exchange of gases in the lungs, while asanas boost blood circulation, ensuring proper oxygen and carbon dioxide levels in every cell.

Ether, or Space This is the almost empty space at the core of matter, as described by quantum physics. It is here that prana (see p178) – invisible vital energy – circulates. Yoga postures allow prana to flow freely and breathing exercises increase its vibratory level.

Benefits for the heart

Modern science is now discovering the many health benefits that classical yoga postures bring to mind and body. Among the most important benefits discovered so far is the effect of yoga on the heart.

All physical exercise promotes better blood circulation and a stronger heart. Although yoga is gentler than most other types of exercise, it still provides a good cardiac workout. In addition, when you practise inverted poses, such as Headstand (see pp62–75) or Shoulderstand (see pp76–9), your heart benefits from a unique form of stimulation.

In these inverted, or upside-down, poses, the pull of gravity draws the blood from the legs and lower trunk back to the heart. This boosted blood flow stretches the heart muscle, which then contracts more powerfully, pumping an increased amount of blood to the whole body.

Blood returns with ease from the body's extremities

Veins return more deoxygenated blood to the heart, from where it returns to the lungs

Arteries carry extra oxygenated blood via the heart around the whole body

Extra blood reaches every cell in the body, reviving and restoring them

Stretched by the boosted blood flow, the heart contracts more powerfully

The brain is bathed in oxygenated blood

INVERSIONS FOR HEALTH
In inverted poses, such as Headstand, there is increased blood flow back to the heart. This gives you an effortless cardiac workout.

Muscles and movement

Asanas promote health by increasing the range of motion in the joints, keeping the body mobile. At most joints, muscles are arranged in opposing pairs; movement takes place when one muscle contracts, or shortens, while the other relaxes and lengthens.

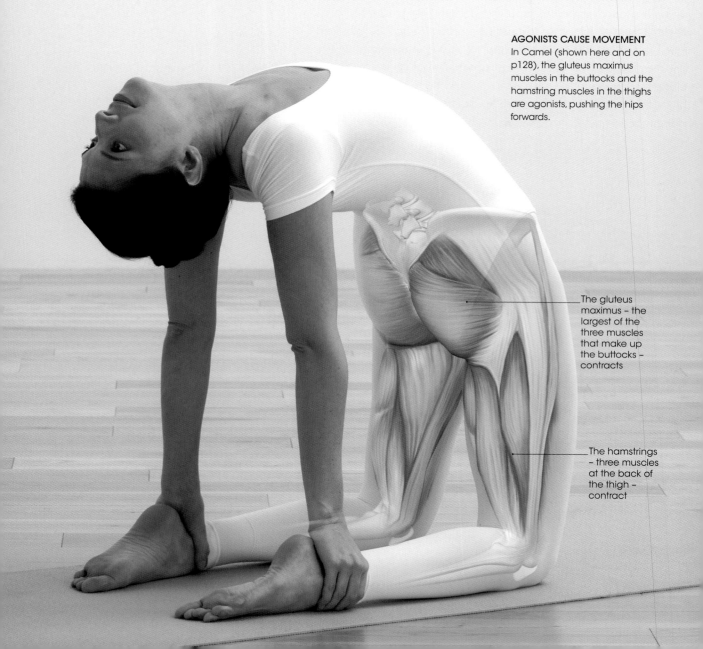

AGONISTS CAUSE MOVEMENT
In Camel (shown here and on p128), the gluteus maximus muscles in the buttocks and the hamstring muscles in the thighs are agonists, pushing the hips forwards.

The gluteus maximus – the largest of the three muscles that make up the buttocks – contracts

The hamstrings – three muscles at the back of the thigh – contract

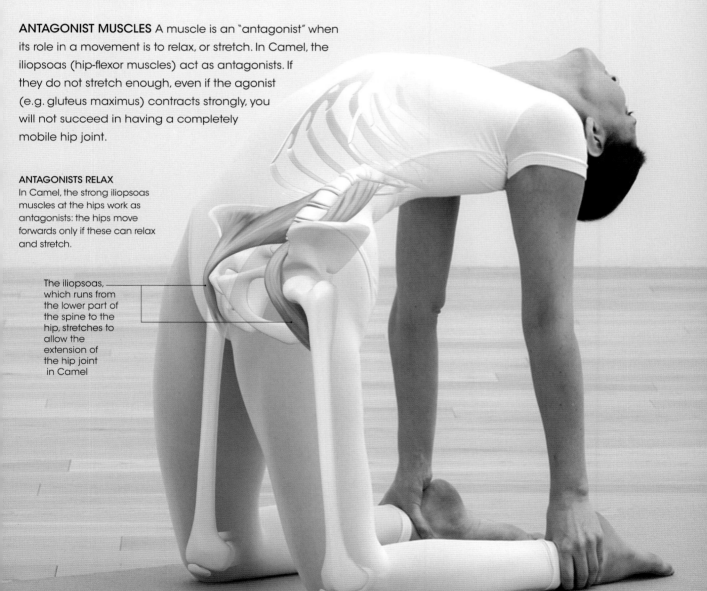

Contraction and relaxation

AGONIST MUSCLES A muscle is called an "agonist" when its contraction causes movement in a joint. For example, in Camel, the contraction of the gluteus maximus acts as an agonist, causing the movement of the thigh in the hip joint. If the gluteus maximus is not strong enough to contract fully, you will lack full range of movement in the hip joint.

ANTAGONIST MUSCLES A muscle is an "antagonist" when its role in a movement is to relax, or stretch. In Camel, the iliopsoas (hip-flexor muscles) act as antagonists. If they do not stretch enough, even if the agonist (e.g. gluteus maximus) contracts strongly, you will not succeed in having a completely mobile hip joint.

ANTAGONISTS RELAX
In Camel, the strong iliopsoas muscles at the hips work as antagonists: the hips move forwards only if these can relax and stretch.

The iliopsoas, which runs from the lower part of the spine to the hip, stretches to allow the extension of the hip joint in Camel

ISOMETRIC CONTRACTION Usually, a muscle shortens when it contracts. But in this form of movement, a muscle contracts without shortening. For example, in the variation Triangle with Bent Knee (see below and p168), the quadriceps (front thigh muscle) of the bent leg contracts strongly. In most cases, this would extend the knee and straighten the leg, but with isometric contraction, the knee remains bent while the thigh muscles contract strongly in order to resist the pull of gravity.

ISOMETRIC RESISTANCE
In this Triangle variation, isometric contraction causes the muscles of the left thigh to resist the pull of gravity, without creating any movement in the knee.

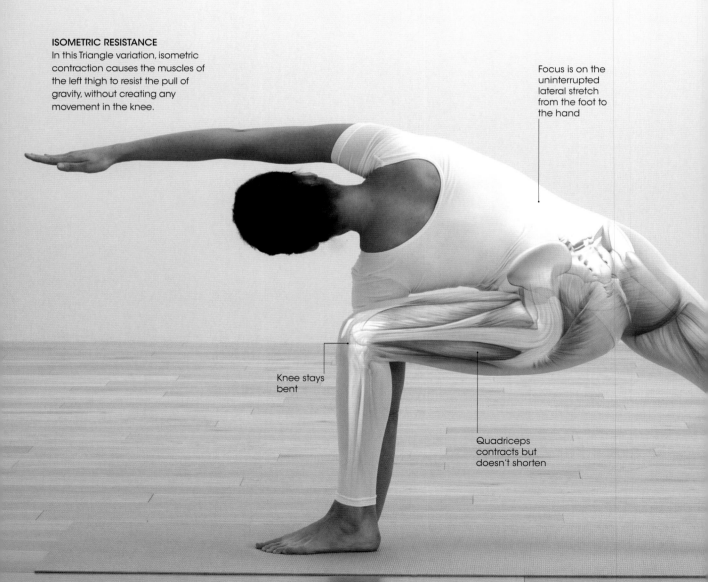

Focus is on the uninterrupted lateral stretch from the foot to the hand

Knee stays bent

Quadriceps contracts but doesn't shorten

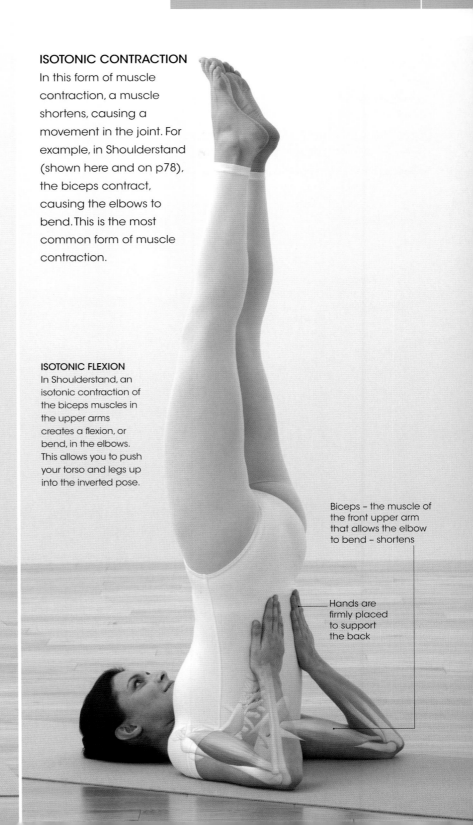

ISOTONIC CONTRACTION

In this form of muscle contraction, a muscle shortens, causing a movement in the joint. For example, in Shoulderstand (shown here and on p78), the biceps contract, causing the elbows to bend. This is the most common form of muscle contraction.

ISOTONIC FLEXION
In Shoulderstand, an isotonic contraction of the biceps muscles in the upper arms creates a flexion, or bend, in the elbows. This allows you to push your torso and legs up into the inverted pose.

Biceps – the muscle of the front upper arm that allows the elbow to bend – shortens

Hands are firmly placed to support the back

Knee straightens

ECCENTRIC CONTRACTION This form of muscular contraction occurs when a muscle contracts and stretches at the same time. In the basic Triangle (shown here and p165), the lateral (sideways) flexion of the spine creates a deep stretch in the iliopsoas muscles in the pelvis. At the same time, the trunk is held parallel to the floor and the lower arm is not allowed to support the body weight. This forces the iliopsoas muscle fibres to contract as they are stretching.

Proper eccentric contraction requires good body awareness, which is one reason why Triangle and its variations are practised at the end of a yoga session.

Stretching the iliopsoas muscle on this side improves the flexibility of the hip joint and the lower back

ECCENTRIC MOVEMENT
In Triangle pose, the upper iliopsoas muscle in the pelvis is being stretched by the lateral movement, while simultaneously contracting to stabilize the asana.

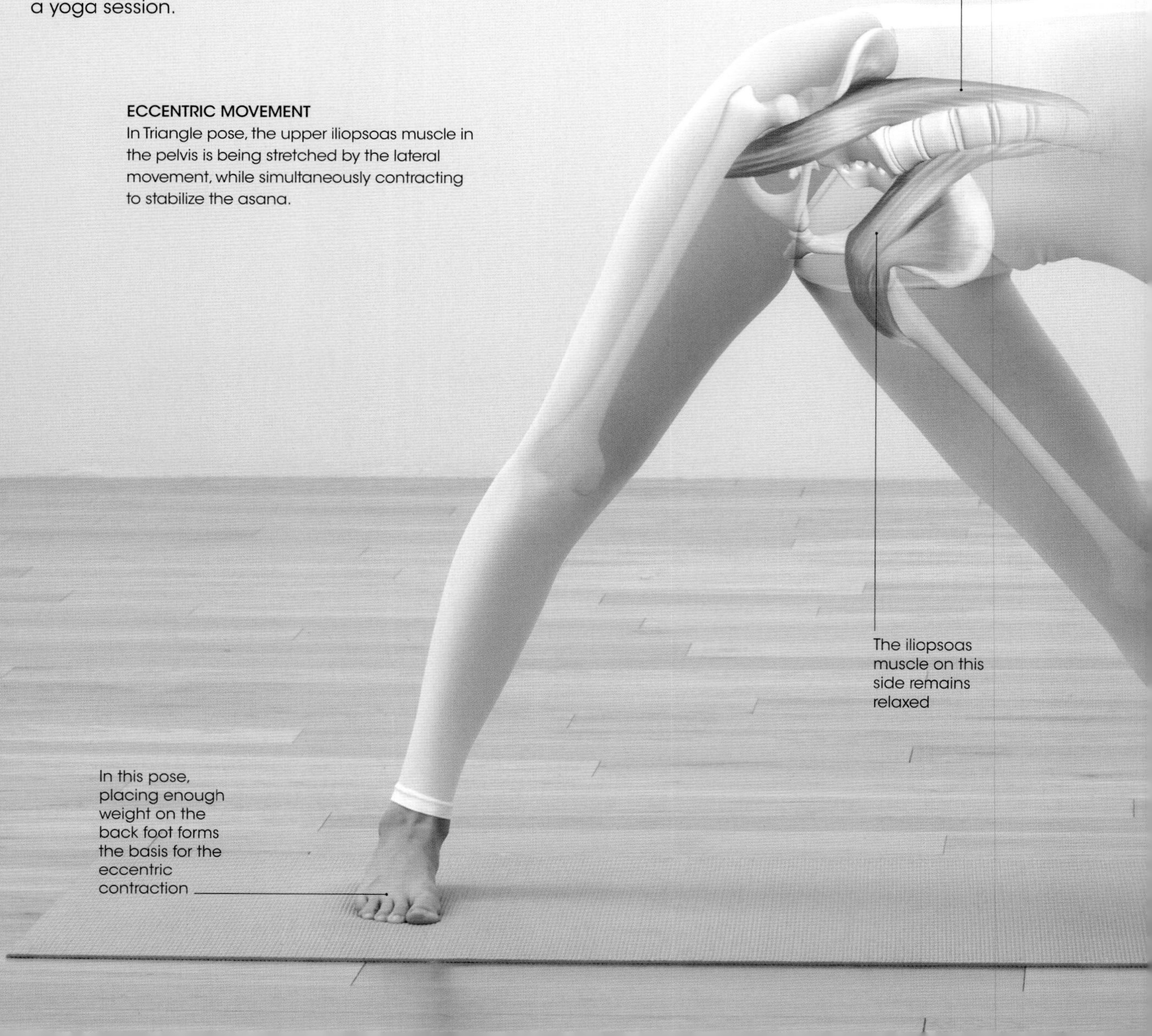

The iliopsoas muscle on this side remains relaxed

In this pose, placing enough weight on the back foot forms the basis for the eccentric contraction

The horizontal position of the torso extends the eccentric contraction all the way from the hip to the shoulder

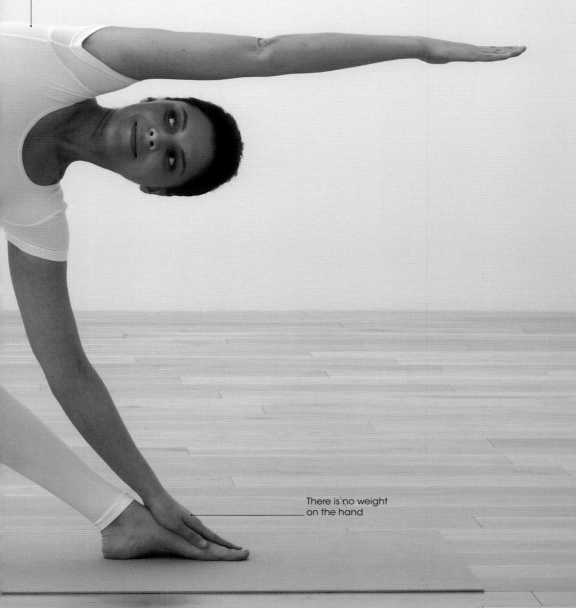

There is no weight on the hand

STRETCHING FROM FOOT TO HEAD Muscles do not only cause or prevent movement in specific joints (see agonist and antagonist, pp20–1). They can also be arranged in long chains, which transmit either a muscle stretch or a muscle contraction from one end of the body to the other. These chains are created by a special form of connective tissue called "fascia". Fascia surrounds every muscle cell and each muscle as a whole. It also connects one muscle with another. Fascia is what allows the powerful, complete stretch along the back of the body in Standing Forward Bend shown here (see also p163). For additional information on connective tissue, see p28.

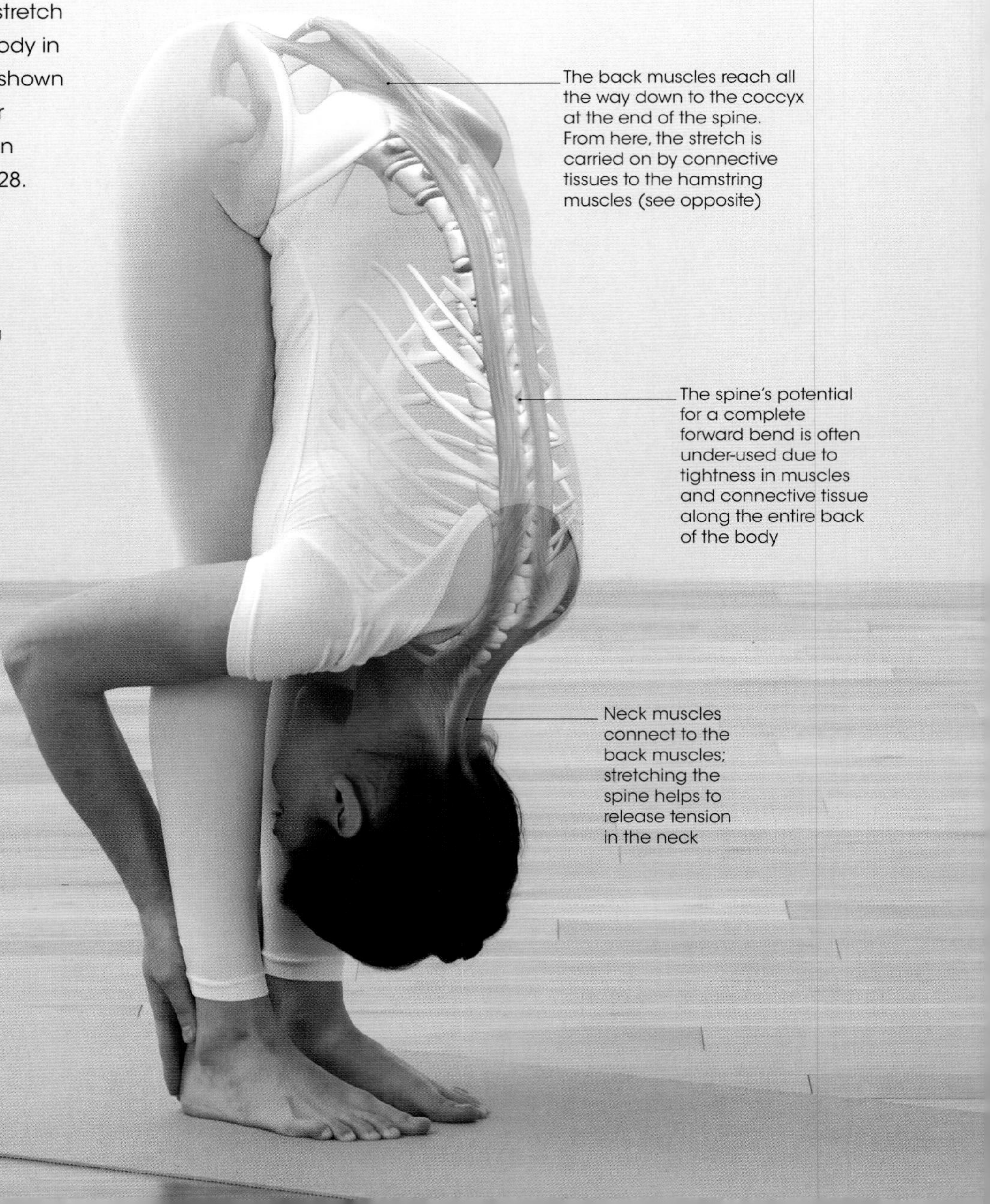

FASCIA IN ACTION
In Standing Forward Bend, the muscles and fascia connect, forming one long chain along the back of the body.

The back muscles reach all the way down to the coccyx at the end of the spine. From here, the stretch is carried on by connective tissues to the hamstring muscles (see opposite)

The spine's potential for a complete forward bend is often under-used due to tightness in muscles and connective tissue along the entire back of the body

Neck muscles connect to the back muscles; stretching the spine helps to release tension in the neck

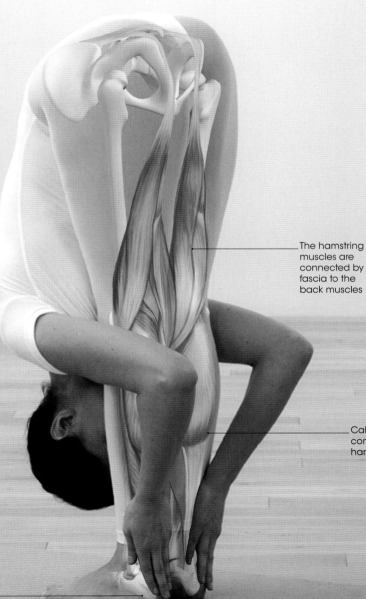

STRETCHING FOR MOBILITY
The Forward Bend stretches the hamstrings, helping to prevent lower back pain. The calf muscles provide "push-off" power for walking; because they are connected, when the hamstrings are stretched, the calf muscles stretch, too, which keeps them supple.

The hamstring muscles are connected by fascia to the back muscles

Calf muscles are connected to the hamstring muscles

Muscles and fascia form a chain from foot to head

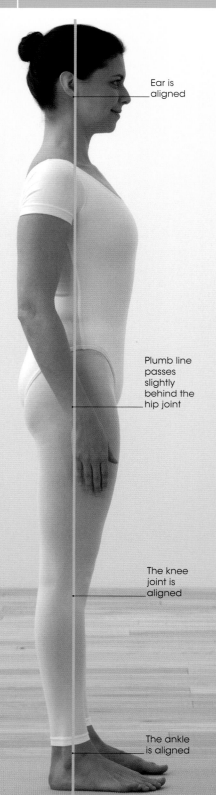

Ear is aligned

Plumb line passes slightly behind the hip joint

The knee joint is aligned

The ankle is aligned

Aligning the posture

Most people don't have well-aligned posture. Practising asanas focuses on strengthening and stretching key muscles. This will help to improve gradually any faulty alignment, particularly in the upper and lower back.

How the body benefits

Aligning your posture involves improving the balance between muscle length and muscle strength. Yoga does this perfectly, because when you hold an asana and then practise its counterpose, the major muscles on the front and back of the body are both stretched and strengthened. This creates tone as well as flexibility. Yoga asanas also have a positive effect on the muscles' connective tissue, or fascia (see pp26–7). Muscles are elastic: after they stretch or contract, the fibres return to their original length. Fascia, however, is plastic not elastic, which means that only if enough pressure is applied, will it change its form and it will not revert to its previous shape when the pressure is removed. Constant repetition of certain movements or body positions, such as always carrying a bag on one shoulder or hunching in front of a computer, fixes the connective tissue into a belt-like, non-elastic structure, causing postural problems. When you hold an asana for longer than a minute, this hardened connective tissue starts to be remodelled, bringing your posture back into proper alignment.

GOOD ALIGNMENT
When someone who has correct posture stands beside a plumb line, the ankles, knees, hips, and ears are aligned perfectly, stacked one above the other in a straight line.

Corrective asanas for kyphosis

Kyphosis, or an exaggerated curve of the spine in the upper back, is a common problem of postural alignment, which is exacerbated by slouching or spending long hours hunching forwards over a computer. These specific asanas gently help to bring the spine into alignment.

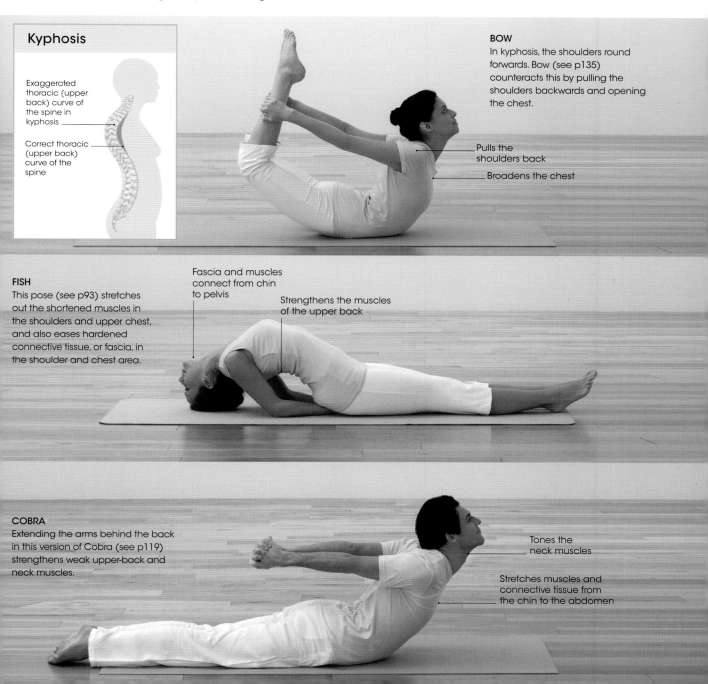

Kyphosis

Exaggerated thoracic (upper back) curve of the spine in kyphosis

Correct thoracic (upper back) curve of the spine

BOW
In kyphosis, the shoulders round forwards. Bow (see p135) counteracts this by pulling the shoulders backwards and opening the chest.

Pulls the shoulders back

Broadens the chest

FISH
This pose (see p93) stretches out the shortened muscles in the shoulders and upper chest, and also eases hardened connective tissue, or fascia, in the shoulder and chest area.

Fascia and muscles connect from chin to pelvis

Strengthens the muscles of the upper back

COBRA
Extending the arms behind the back in this version of Cobra (see p119) strengthens weak upper-back and neck muscles.

Tones the neck muscles

Stretches muscles and connective tissue from the chin to the abdomen

Corrective asanas for lordosis

In this condition, the muscles of the abdomen tend to be weak, and the hamstrings and lower back muscles have become shortened. Connective tissue (see pp26–7) along the back of the legs and back has hardened. These poses help to strengthen and lengthen the muscles and soften the tissue.

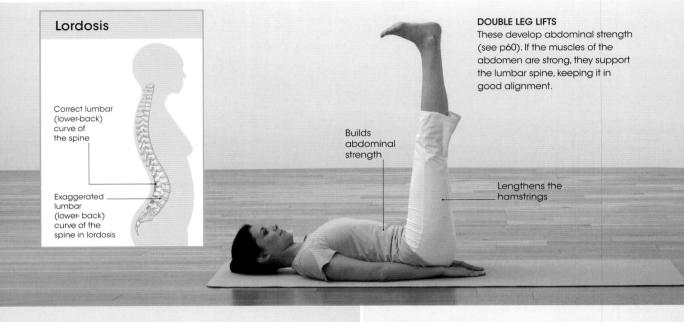

Lordosis

Correct lumbar (lower-back) curve of the spine

Exaggerated lumbar (lower- back) curve of the spine in lordosis

DOUBLE LEG LIFTS
These develop abdominal strength (see p60). If the muscles of the abdomen are strong, they support the lumbar spine, keeping it in good alignment.

Builds abdominal strength

Lengthens the hamstrings

SITTING FORWARD BEND

This pose (see p99) gives a deep stretch to the muscles of the back of the body, which have become shortened. Try to hold the pose for some time, stretching slowly and gradually. As long as any pain that comes from the natural stretch can be dissolved by rhythmical abdominal breathing and relaxation, it is safe to remain in the posture. Any other pain should be taken as a warning sign not to take the stretch too far.

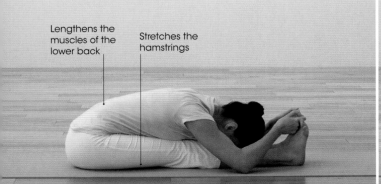

Lengthens the muscles of the lower back

Stretches the hamstrings

STANDING FORWARD BEND

Another stretch to lengthen the whole of the back of the body (see p163). As you stretch, use slow, controlled breathing and consciously relax. This, together with repeated practice, will ease any pain and boost flexibility.

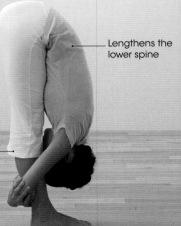

Lengthens the lower spine

Stretches the backs of the legs

Corrective asanas for scoliosis

When the spinal muscles diagonally opposite each other are shortened on one side and overstretched on the other, it leads to scoliosis. For example, the left side of the lumbar and the right side of the thoracic spine could be pulled out of alignment. Holding asanas to the right and left rebalances the muscles.

Scoliosis

Lateral (side to side) deviation of the spine in scoliosis

Correct position of the spine

HALF SPINAL TWIST
Hold this pose (see p148), and all other poses on this page, for the same length of time on each side. This ensures stretching and strengthening in all the required areas.

Increases flexibility on one side

Tones the muscles on the other side

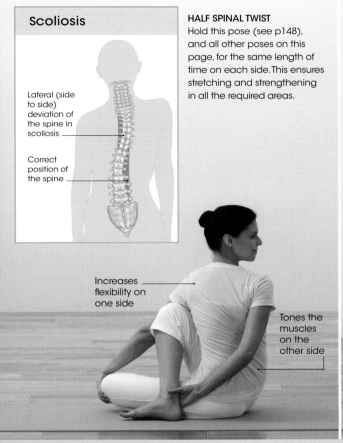

TRIANGLE
Asanas such as Triangle (see p165) that are practised to the right and left sides restore the correct balance of flexibility and strength to the muscles on either side of the spine. They also help to soften hardened connective tissue.

Stretches the muscles on the right side

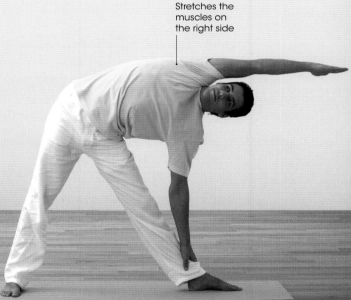

LATERAL BEND WITH TWIST
Lateral stretches such as Lateral Bend with Twist (see p107) help to restore the balance of shortened muscles on diagonally opposite sides of the spine. Always move slowly into the pose to overcome gradually any inherent resistance in the muscles.

Stretches from hip to shoulder

The breath of life

Breathing is like no other body function because it connects us with our environment. Plants take in carbon dioxide and give off oxygen, while human beings and animals inhale oxygen-rich air and exhale air high in carbon dioxide. Yoga breathing exercises help to increase the gas exchange in the lungs and in all the cells of the body.

Involuntary breathing

Most of the time we breathe involuntarily, thanks to respiratory-control centres located in the brain. An average adult respiratory rate varies between 12 and 20 breaths per minute at rest, moving about half a litre (1 pint) of air in and out of the lungs – this is the vital capacity. When an adult exercises, the respiratory rate can go up to 35–45 breaths per minute, increasing vital capacity to over 4 litres (8½ pints) of inhaled and exhaled air. Such fast, deep breathing is prompted by a sudden increase in carbon-dioxide waste in the muscles caused by exercising.

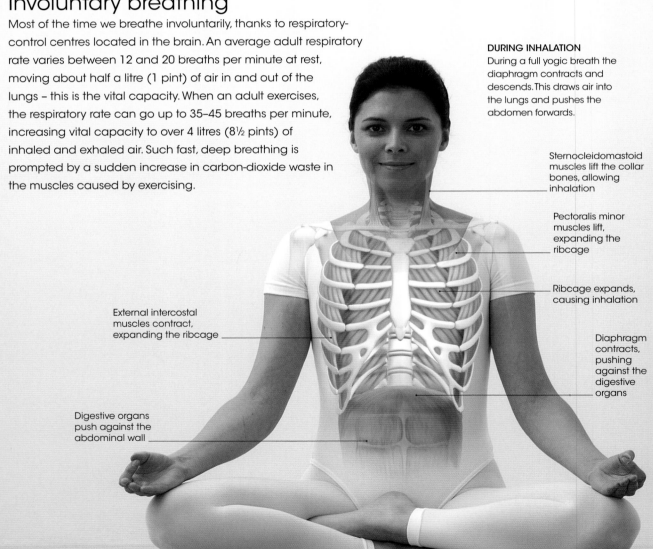

DURING INHALATION
During a full yogic breath the diaphragm contracts and descends. This draws air into the lungs and pushes the abdomen forwards.

Sternocleidomastoid muscles lift the collar bones, allowing inhalation

Pectoralis minor muscles lift, expanding the ribcage

Ribcage expands, causing inhalation

Diaphragm contracts, pushing against the digestive organs

External intercostal muscles contract, expanding the ribcage

Digestive organs push against the abdominal wall

Voluntary breath control

Yoga emphasizes voluntary breath control. During asana practice, breathing slows to 10–12 breaths per minute. In relaxation and meditation, you breathe only 6–8 times per minute, and you take just 3–6 breaths per minute during Alternate Nostril Breathing (see pp182–3). All respiratory training in yoga emphasizes complete exhalation in order to eliminate maximum amounts of stale air and allow a deeper inhalation.

In this way, freshly inhaled oxygen-rich air mixes with lesser amounts of stale air than in involuntary breathing, making more oxygen available to nourish every cell. During pranayama, oxygen levels in the blood are higher when you inhale and much lower when you retain your breath. Studies by the Russian medical researcher Dr Arkadi F. Prokop suggest that exposure to alternating high and low levels of oxygen promotes cell rejuvenation, speeding up the renewal of mitochondria – the microscopic power plants in every cell. Many asanas create pressure on the chest and abdomen. Performing a complete yogic breath (see p181) against such resistance strengthens the respiratory muscles and helps you to breathe with greater awareness in daily life.

DURING EXHALATION
The diaphragm relaxes and moves up, pushing air out of the lungs and allowing the abdomen to move back in.

Sternocleidomastoid muscles relax

Pectoralis minor muscles relax, so the chest drops

External intercostal muscles relax, so the chest sinks

Diaphragm relaxes

Abdominal muscles contract, pushing internal organs against the diaphragm for complete exhalation

Supporting the nervous system

Yoga works on the nervous system, keeping it in balance so that you feel better able to deal with the unavoidable stresses that are part of daily life. The order of the 12 basic poses (see pp42–169) and the focus on posture, breathing, and relaxation in each asana help the nervous system function, leading to a sense of complete relaxation and rejuvenation.

What is the autonomic nervous system?

The autonomic nervous system fine-tunes the activities of the vital organs of the body, such as the heart, as well as the respiratory, digestive, and endocrine systems (see p37). It also governs homeostasis (see p18). This system functions involuntarily, ensuring that nerves transmit messages between the brain and organs, muscles, and glands, through the central nervous system in the brain and spinal cord. The autonomic nervous system is divided into two: the sympathetic and parasympathetic systems.

THE SYMPATHETIC NERVOUS SYSTEM This branch of the autonomic nervous system sends out nerve impulses, in response to perceived physical or psychological danger, that trigger the release of hormones including adrenaline and noradrenaline. These prepare the body for fighting the danger or fleeing from it (the "fight or flight response") by stimulating an increase in heart rate and blood pressure, diverting blood to the skeletal muscles, and slowing the digestion and kidney function, among other reactions. These stress responses continue until the body fights or runs away or the parasympathetic nervous system becomes dominant. If the responses are not dispelled, over time they can damage the body and mind.

THE PARASYMPATHETIC NERVOUS SYSTEM The other branch of the autonomic nervous system promotes rest, energy conservation, and the absorption of nutrients to maintain good health. It also supports the regular functioning of the cardiovascular, digestive, and excretory systems among other vital processes, and acts as an antidote to the "fight or flight" response. Practising yoga asanas (see pp42–169), pranayama (see pp176–85), and meditation (see pp196–207) activates this "rest and repair" branch of the autonomic nervous system.

Sympathetic and parasympathetic activity

The two systems work in a complementary way. As the brain anticipates danger, the sympathetic neurons in the spinal cord release chemical nerve transmitters. These trigger target organs, muscles, and glands to prepare to deal with stress by reacting as shown below. When the parasympathic nerves are stimulated, they gradually cancel these responses.

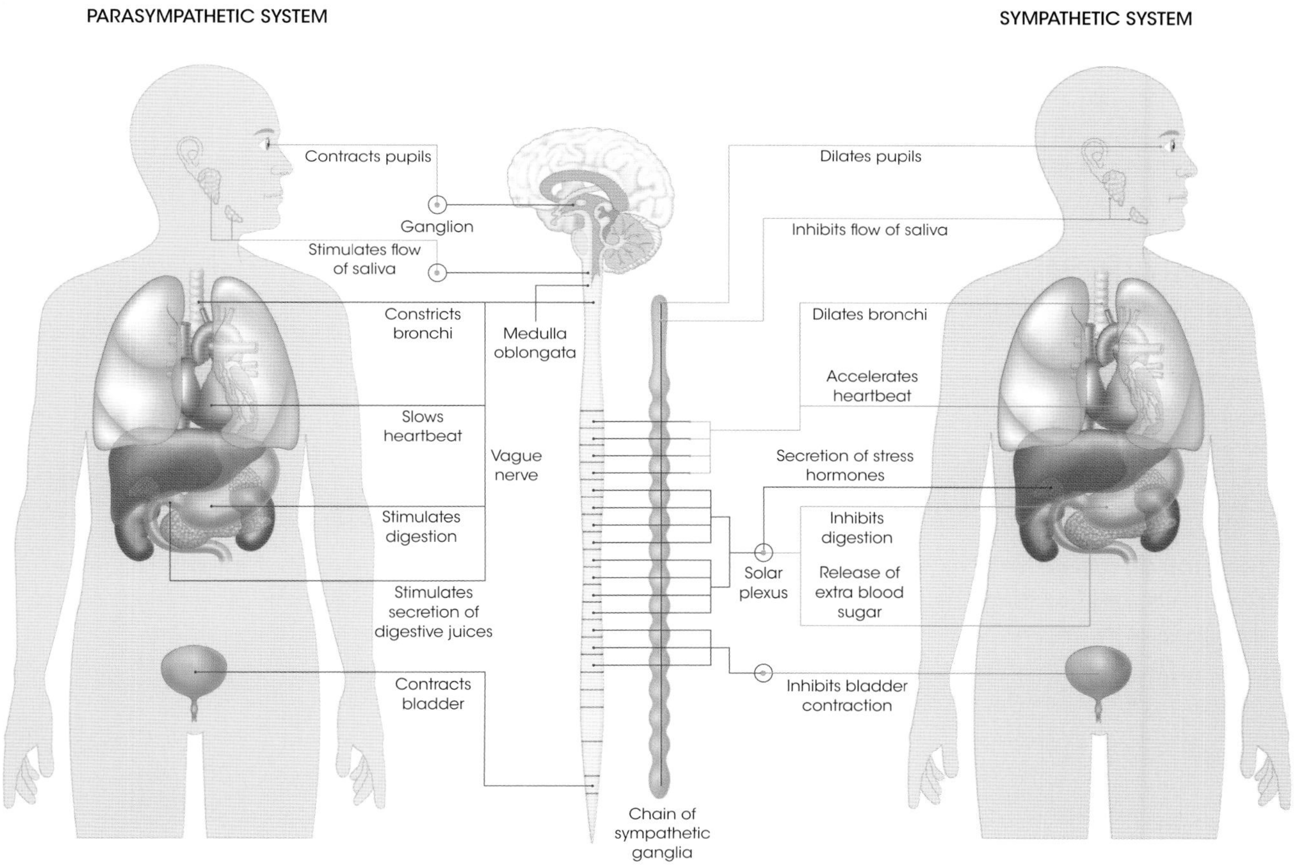

PARASYMPATHETIC SYSTEM

SYMPATHETIC SYSTEM

Contracts pupils

Dilates pupils

Ganglion

Inhibits flow of saliva

Stimulates flow of saliva

Constricts bronchi

Medulla oblongata

Dilates bronchi

Accelerates heartbeat

Slows heartbeat

Vague nerve

Secretion of stress hormones

Stimulates digestion

Inhibits digestion

Solar plexus

Release of extra blood sugar

Stimulates secretion of digestive juices

Contracts bladder

Inhibits bladder contraction

Chain of sympathetic ganglia

THE AUTONOMIC NERVOUS SYSTEM
The sympathetic system is important because it primes us to deal with stressful situations, promoting alertness and quick-thinking. When the parasympathetic system is in action after a period of sympathetic activity, it provides optimum conditions for good health.

Yoga to balance the nervous system

Structuring your asana practice in the following way can help to restore the balance between the sympathetic and parasympathetic nervous systems.

SUN SALUTATION At the beginning of your asana session, practise Sun Salutations (see pp50–7) to start reducing sympathetic nerve impulses.

ALTERNATE MUSCLE STRETCHING AND RELAXATION Then practise asanas that focus mostly on flexibility (see pp58–115), followed by appropriate relaxation poses. Alternating the slight muscle pain of stretching with relaxation stimulates the parasympathetic nervous system, helping you to relax.

ALTERNATE MUSCLE CONTRACTION AND RELAXATION Now you will do mostly short, intense muscle contractions (see pp116–69), followed by conscious relaxation to prompt "rest and repair" impulses in the parasympathetic system.

FINAL RELAXATION During final relaxation (see pp192–3), your body is flooded with parasympathetic nerve impulses. When you return to a stressful environment your sympathetic nerve impulses may be stimulated again, but thanks to the strength of the parasympathetic "rest and repair" impulses you experience in your asana practice, they will have little effect on you.

Muscle stretching and relaxation

Notice how any pain you feel in the muscles during the stretches disappears completely during the complementary relaxation pose. You are literally stretching the stress away.

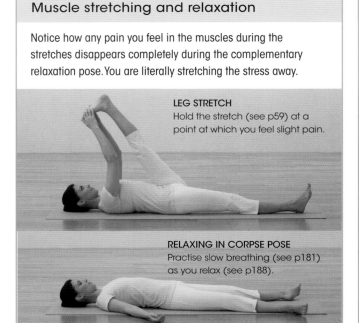

LEG STRETCH
Hold the stretch (see p59) at a point at which you feel slight pain.

RELAXING IN CORPSE POSE
Practise slow breathing (see p181) as you relax (see p188).

Muscle contraction and relaxation

Some asanas demand more dynamic muscle work. When followed immediately by an appropriate relaxation pose, you stimulate the parasympathetic nervous system.

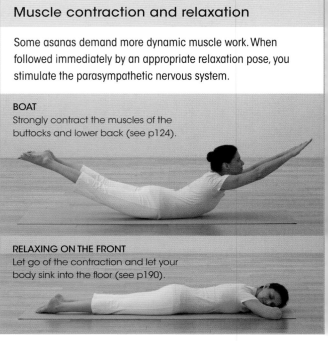

BOAT
Strongly contract the muscles of the buttocks and lower back (see p124).

RELAXING ON THE FRONT
Let go of the contraction and let your body sink into the floor (see p190).

Yoga and the endocrine system

The endocrine glands secrete hormones into the blood stream. These chemical "messengers" reach every cell of the body. They initiate and regulate many body functions. Yoga helps to keep this body system in good shape.

What does it do?

The main endocrine gland is the pituitary gland in the brain. Other glands include the pineal, also in the brain, which produces melatonin to control the sleep-wake cycle, and the thyroid in the neck, which releases hormones regulating growth and metabolism. At the back of this gland is the parathyroid, which promotes calcium absorption. The thymus at the top of the chest regulates immunity; the adrenals on top of each kidney oversee fluid balance, fat distribution, and stress hormones. The pancreas, an organ, regulates blood-sugar levels and the ovaries or testes release sex hormones.

Benefits for the brain

Practising asanas helps to bring balance to the brain and, through the pituitary gland, to the whole body. In certain asanas, such as Headstand, extra blood circulates to the brain, nourishing it with oxygen and nutrients. This improves the working of the hypothalamus.

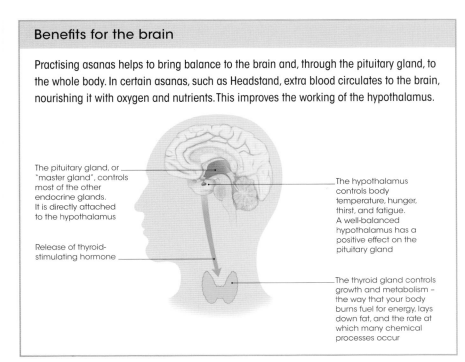

The pituitary gland, or "master gland", controls most of the other endocrine glands. It is directly attached to the hypothalamus

Release of thyroid-stimulating hormone

The hypothalamus controls body temperature, hunger, thirst, and fatigue. A well-balanced hypothalamus has a positive effect on the pituitary gland

The thyroid gland controls growth and metabolism – the way that your body burns fuel for energy, lays down fat, and the rate at which many chemical processes occur

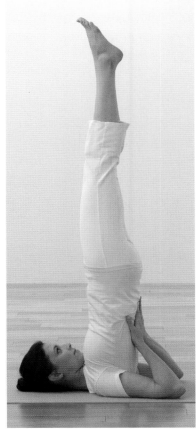

SHOULDERSTAND
When you hold this pose (see p78), you increase the blood circulation in the thyroid gland in the neck, which promotes a healthy metabolism.

Yoga and relaxation

Yoga teaches you how to achieve deep muscle relaxation, first by following a muscle contraction in one asana with complete muscular relaxation in its complementary resting pose. Second, by using autosuggestion in final relaxation (see pp192–4), asking each part of the body in turn to relax until you experience a feeling of total release.

A strong muscle contraction requires a large number of nerve impulses to command muscle fibres to shorten; complete relaxation requires the fewest nerve impulses to be directed to the fibres. These processes seem opposed, but the more you relax before moving into an asana, the more efficiently you will be able to focus on muscle contraction, and the deeper you will be able to breathe. Follow the asana with its relaxation pose; then the complete release of the contraction plus slow breathing stimulates deep relaxation.

Using autosuggestion

To achieve deep muscle relaxation in final relaxation (see pp192–4), lie comfortably, then create a mental picture of the muscles of the body in turn, and send them a mental command to relax, which travels via impulses from the motor cortex in the brain. The command is followed quickly by a feeling of relaxation.

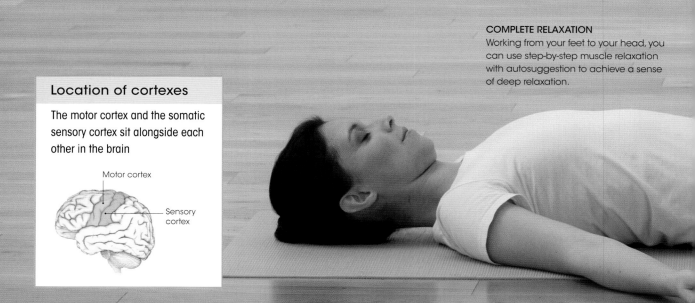

COMPLETE RELAXATION
Working from your feet to your head, you can use step-by-step muscle relaxation with autosuggestion to achieve a sense of deep relaxation.

Location of cortexes

The motor cortex and the somatic sensory cortex sit alongside each other in the brain

Motor cortex

Sensory cortex

Brain mapping

The sequence of autosuggestion during relaxation is "mapped" in the motor cortex (see location in the brain, opposite). The sensation of relaxation that follows corresponds to the "map" of the somatic sensory cortex. Although there is no direct motor control to the intra-abdominal organs, the autosuggestion reaches the target organ via the subconscious mind.

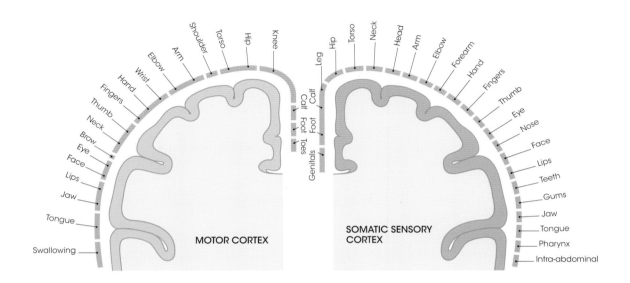

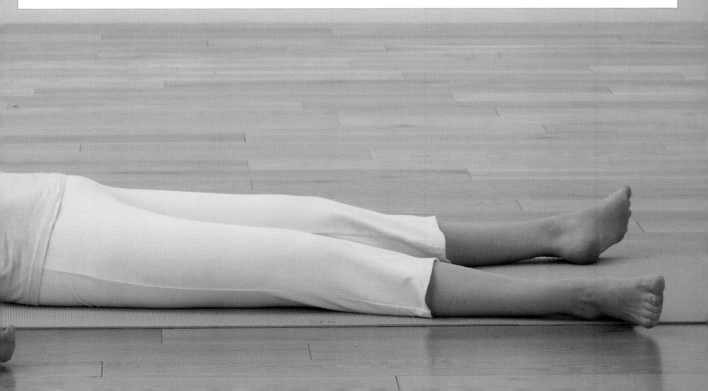

One pose, many benefits

Asanas work on many body systems simultaneously. Gaining a better understanding of how some of these benefits complement each other can bring you one step closer to understanding the Sanskrit word *yoga*, which translates as "union". Here, we look at the benefits a single asana can bring to many parts of the body and the mind.

Effects on the body

Practising this variation of Triangle pose (see p167) benefits all ten body systems, from the skeletal to the reproductive, but these in particular:

MUSCULAR SYSTEM The muscles at the front of the thighs contract to keep the leg stable, while those at the back of the thighs extend. Balancing muscle strength with length maintains mobility in the joints. Repeating the pose to both sides promotes good posture by working the spine evenly.

NERVOUS SYSTEM The spine, containing the central nervous system, receives a good stretch along its length, which benefits communication between the spinal nerves and the brain. The cerebellum controls smooth movement, proper alignment, and stable posture.

ENDOCRINE SYSTEM Blood flows easily to the brain in this pose, supporting the pituitary gland (see p37), which regulates hormone secretion throughout the body. More specifically, the pressure of the pose stimulates the adrenal gland. This helps to ensure its role in the "fight or flight response" (see p34) and in processing food and regulating energy.

DIGESTIVE SYSTEM As the trunk revolves, the digestive organs receive a massage, which stimulates the functioning of the digestive system. The pressure on the organs pushes stagnating blood out of them, which in turn draws fresh blood supply into this area, once the pose is released.

CARDIOVASCULAR AND RESPIRATORY SYSTEMS This pose requires some exertion, working the muscles of the heart and increasing the lungs' vital capacity (see p32-3). The respiratory muscles also get a good workout from working against the compression of the twist. Both actions ensure a good supply of oxygen to the brain, encouraging concentration and vitality.

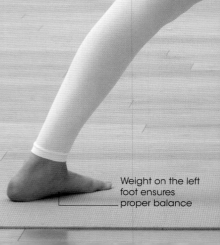

Weight on the left foot ensures proper balance

Massage of the adrenal glands helps deal with stress

Massage of the digestive system makes it work more efficiently

Eccentric muscle contraction on the left side of the back keeps the torso aligned horizontally

The left hip rotates inwards

The hamstring muscles of the right leg stretch deeply

The right hip rotates outwards

What happens in the brain

The pose activates the cerebellum to maintain balance. It also massages the adrenal glands on top of the kidneys, whose function is controlled by the pituitary gland in the brain.

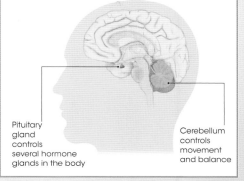

Pituitary gland controls several hormone glands in the body

Cerebellum controls movement and balance

Rotation of the spine tones the spinal nerves and improves their communication with the brain

The cerebellum is stimulated into controlling balance

The pituitary gland controls the secretions of the adrenal gland

TRIANGLE POSE
As well as the benefits on the various body systems, this asana enhances balance and spatial awareness.

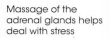

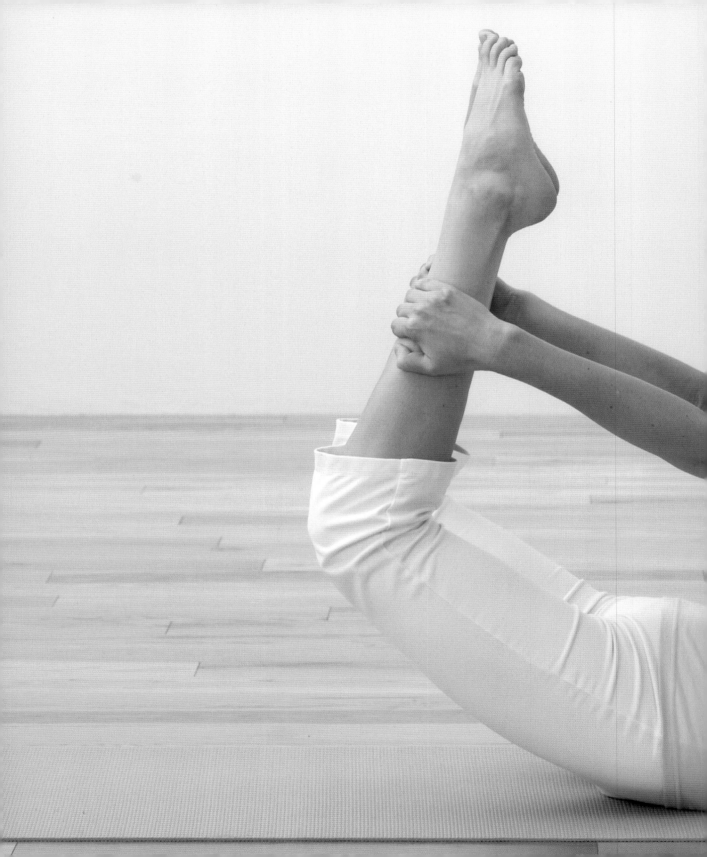

Proper Exercise

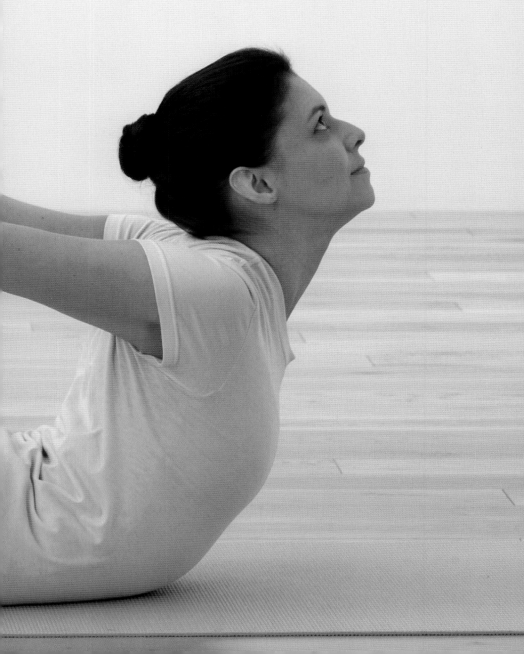

What is proper exercise?

The twelve basic postures, or asanas, should be practiced in a specific order. The aim is to promote good health and to awaken the subtle energy – prana (see p178) – in your body. After you have finished your yoga practice, you will feel a profound sense of physical and emotional wellbeing.

A logical sequence

The sequence of twelve basic asanas are specially designed to help your body and mind to reap the greatest possible benefits. They should be followed in the order given in this book and you should practise them at every session. Also take care to follow any breathing instructions given as well as the guidelines for relaxation poses in between asanas.

INITIAL RELAXATION Always begin with relaxation in Corpse Pose (see p46) to focus your mind and prevent you from being distracted by the demands of everyday life. Continue with Easy Sitting Pose (see p47). This gives you a firm sitting position for performing the Eye and Neck Exercises (see pp48–9), as well as the breathing exercises (see pp180–5). Next comes the Sun Salutation (see pp50–7), which stimulates the heart and the circulation of the blood. It also serves as a general warm-up for the poses that follow.

THE FIRST HALF OF YOUR PRACTICE After the Sun Salutation, you move on to asanas that focus mostly on muscle stretching. The stretching is always followed by relaxation of the muscles. In addition, the inverted poses of this first part of your practice increase the blood supply to the head, which improves the function of the brain and the thyroid gland.

THE SECOND HALF OF YOUR PRACTICE From Cobra onwards (see p116), the asanas focus more on muscle strengthening. This is done by contracting then relaxing the muscles. In addition, poses such as Bow (see pp134–43), Half Spinal Twist (see pp144–9), and Peacock (see pp154–61) exert more pressure on your inner organs. This helps to detoxify the tissues and increase their blood supply.

FINAL RELAXATION Practise final relaxation lying in Corpse Pose (see pp192–3). Never omit this essential part of your practice. When you relax in this position, your voluntary muscles and your internal organs relax completely. Final relaxation also helps you to absorb all the benefits of the asanas you have just practised.

When to practice

You can schedule your yoga practice anytime from early morning to late evening. The most important considerations are:

• You should not eat 2–3 hours before you practise.

• Except late in the evening, you should have a wholesome meal or snack shortly after you practise.

• Taking a shower before you practise is advantageous, but a shower is not recommended immediately after, as it neutralises prana (see p178).

• Choose a time when you will not be distracted by phone calls.

From beginner to advanced

The step-by-step instructions in this book guide you from beginner level, through intermediate to advanced. If you are a beginner, you may find that, to start with, you can only manage a few of the steps leading up to the final pose. If this is the case, do not worry and do not force yourself on to the next step. It is not a competition. In yoga, there are benefits for mind and body at every step. When you reach the final pose, look at the illustration showing the common faults in the pose. You may be doing some or all of these. As you practise the pose, try and be aware of your mistakes and do your best to correct them.

Pose and counterpose

Many poses have a counterpose – one that moves the spine and other joints in the opposite direction. So, having performed Shoulderstand (see pp76–8), which gives you a forward bend, Fish (see pp92–3), which is another basic asana in its own right, provides you with a backward bend a little later on in your practice.

Clothing and equipment

Loose cotton clothing that enables you to move easily is ideal. You will also need a rubber mat for practising asanas, and a pillow when you practise the easy sitting position (see p47). You may also like to cover yourself with a thin blanket during final relaxation (see pp192–3).

THE ASANAS AND THEIR VARIATIONS
Most of the twelve basic asanas also have variations. Some variations are poses in their own right, such as Wheel (see pp140–3). Other variations lead on from the basic pose, but take you into more advanced positions, such as this Shoulderstand variation, Arms on Floor (see p79).

Initial Relaxation

Each step of your yoga session demands a fine-tuning of your nervous system. That is why you should always prepare yourself for your asana practice with at least five minutes of complete

Corpse Pose

Lie flat on your back with your arms and legs apart and your eyes closed. Shake out your shoulders to release any tension in them. Slowly roll your head from side to side a couple of times, lowering one ear towards the ground, then the other. Bring your head back to the centre. Lie still as you concentrate on your breath, using the deep abdominal breathing technique described below.

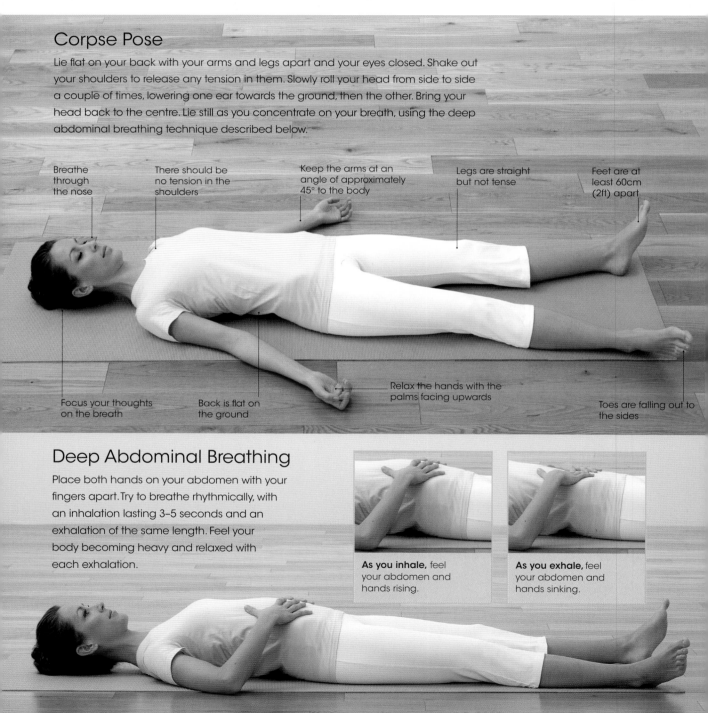

Breathe through the nose

There should be no tension in the shoulders

Keep the arms at an angle of approximately 45° to the body

Legs are straight but not tense

Feet are at least 60cm (2ft) apart

Focus your thoughts on the breath

Back is flat on the ground

Relax the hands with the palms facing upwards

Toes are falling out to the sides

Deep Abdominal Breathing

Place both hands on your abdomen with your fingers apart. Try to breathe rhythmically, with an inhalation lasting 3–5 seconds and an exhalation of the same length. Feel your body becoming heavy and relaxed with each exhalation.

As you inhale, feel your abdomen and hands rising.

As you exhale, feel your abdomen and hands sinking.

relaxation in Corpse Pose, using Deep Abdominal Breathing. Following that, sit in Easy Sitting Pose for 2 minutes, in readiness for the Eye and Neck Exercises (see pp48–9).

Easy Sitting Pose

Sit in a simple, cross-legged position to prepare for the Eye and Neck exercises. This position gives you a very firm, stable base and helps to keep your energy centred.

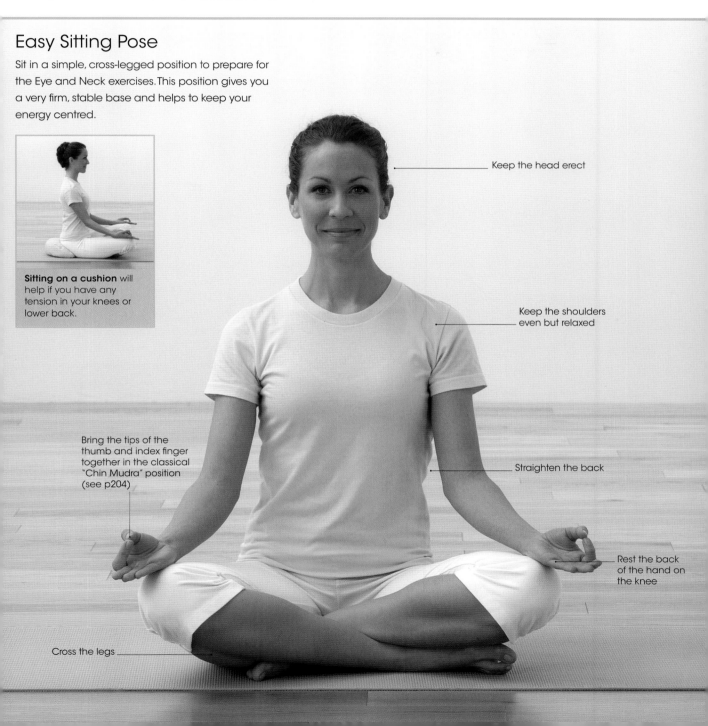

Sitting on a cushion will help if you have any tension in your knees or lower back.

Keep the head erect

Keep the shoulders even but relaxed

Bring the tips of the thumb and index finger together in the classical "Chin Mudra" position (see p204)

Straighten the back

Rest the back of the hand on the knee

Cross the legs

Eye Exercises

In our modern world, the eyes are subjected daily to computer and TV screens, fast-moving traffic, and artificial light. Yogic eye exercises are both relaxing and strengthening for the eyes.

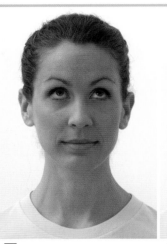 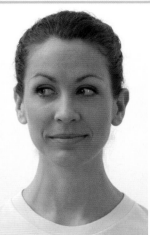 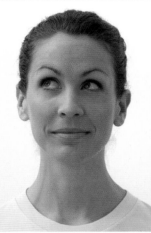 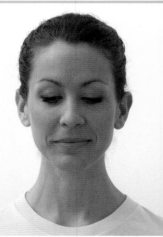

1 Keeping your back and neck straight and your head still, look upwards as high as you can, and then look downwards. Repeat at least 10 times, then close and relax your eyes for about 30 seconds.

2 Opening your eyes wide, look as far to the right as you can, and then look to the left. Repeat at least 10 times, then close and relax your eyes for 30 seconds.

3 Move your eyes diagonally by looking from the upper right-hand corner to the lower left and back again. Repeat 10 times, then repeat the exercise by looking from the top left corner to the bottom right. Close and relax the eyes.

4 Roll your eyes clockwise in wide circles. Start slowly and gradually increase speed until you are moving your eyes as fast as you can. Make at least 10 circles, then close your eyes for a moment. Now repeat counter-clockwise. Close and relax your eyes.

Relaxing the eyes

To soothe and relax your eyes after the exercises, use warm hands cupped over your eyes to provide heat and darkness.

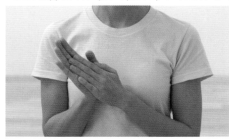 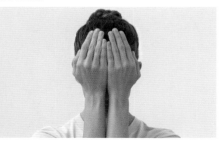

WARMING THE HANDS
When you have finished the eye exercises, rub your hands together vigorously until the friction between them warms up your palms.

CUPPING THE EYES
Gently cup your hands over your closed eyes, without touching the eyelids. Keep them there for about 30 seconds.

Neck Exercises

These exercises aim to release any tension in the neck, shoulders, and upper back. While performing these exercises, only move your head and neck, not your back and shoulders.

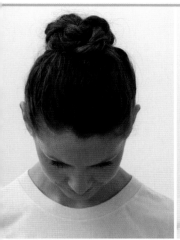 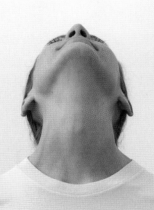 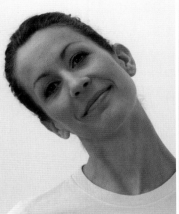 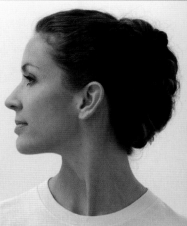

1 Start in the Easy Sitting Position (see p47), with your back straight and your chest erect. Slowly bring your head forwards towards the chest to give the back of your neck a good stretch.

2 After a few moments slowly lift your head and extend your neck as far back as possible.

3 Lower your right ear close to your right shoulder, then repeat on the other side. Keep both shoulders level throughout. Repeat the exercise 5–10 times.

4 Turn your head to the right side. Contract the muscles on the right side of your neck, and feel the stretch on the left side. Repeat on the opposite side. Repeat the exercise 5–10 times.

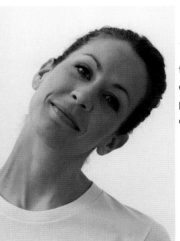

5 Drop your chin to the chest and rotate your head clockwise 2–3 times. Bring your head to the centre and start again, performing 2–3 times in a counter-clockwise direction.

CAUTION Some people cannot extend their neck far. If you feel any dizziness or too much pressure on your neck, extend less until you feel comfortable. Repeat the exercise 5–10 times.

Sun Salutation
All Levels

At the start of Sun Salutation, you need to be standing at the front of your mat. This leaves room behind you for the subsequent steps. Observe how the movements involve counter-stretches –

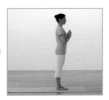 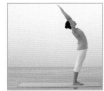 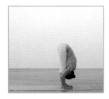 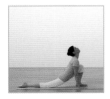 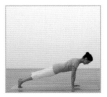 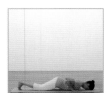

BENEFITS

PHYSICAL
- Gently increases the blood circulation.
- Thoroughly recharges the solar plexus despite being a physical workout.
- Stretches and strengthens dozens of muscles throughout the body.
- Quickly brings flexibility to the spine and the limbs.
- Regulates the breathing.
- Increases the respiratory capacity.

MENTAL
- Gives a clear sense of being in one place in the present moment, thanks to its symmetrical, circular sequence of movements.
- Looking up and down into space allows the mind to expand.
- The increased and detailed body awareness brings greater detachment. The body is seen as the vehicle of the mind and the soul.

1 Exhale as you bring your palms together in front of your chest in Prayer Position.

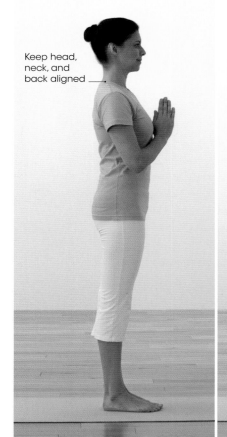

Keep head, neck, and back aligned

Transition to Step 2
Start to inhale as you stretch your arms up next to your ears, palms facing forwards. Avoid tension in the neck as you raise your shoulders.

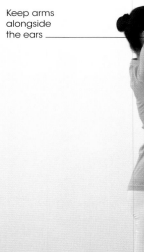

Keep arms alongside the ears

a backward bend followed by a forward bend, which is followed by another backward bend. These movements promote great flexibility in the spine and are beneficial to all levels of practitioner.

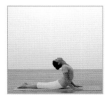 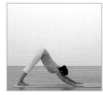 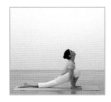 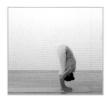 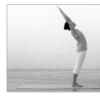 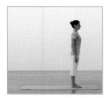

2 As you continue inhaling, take the weight onto your heels, look upwards, and arch your arms, head, and chest backwards. Stretch your chest and abdomen.

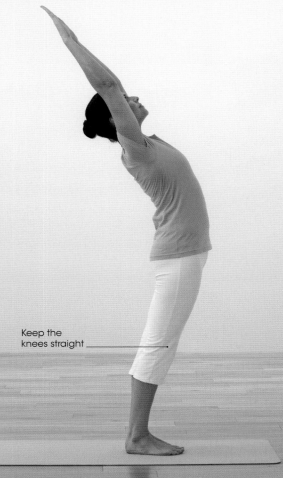

Keep the knees straight

Transition to Step 3

Start to exhale as you bend forwards from the waist, keeping your legs straight. Use your back muscles to bring your spine, head, and arms into a horizontal line.

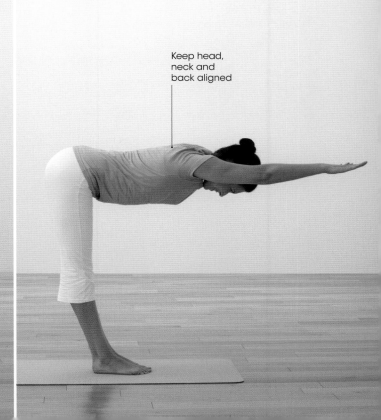

Keep head, neck and back aligned

Sun Salutation
(continued)

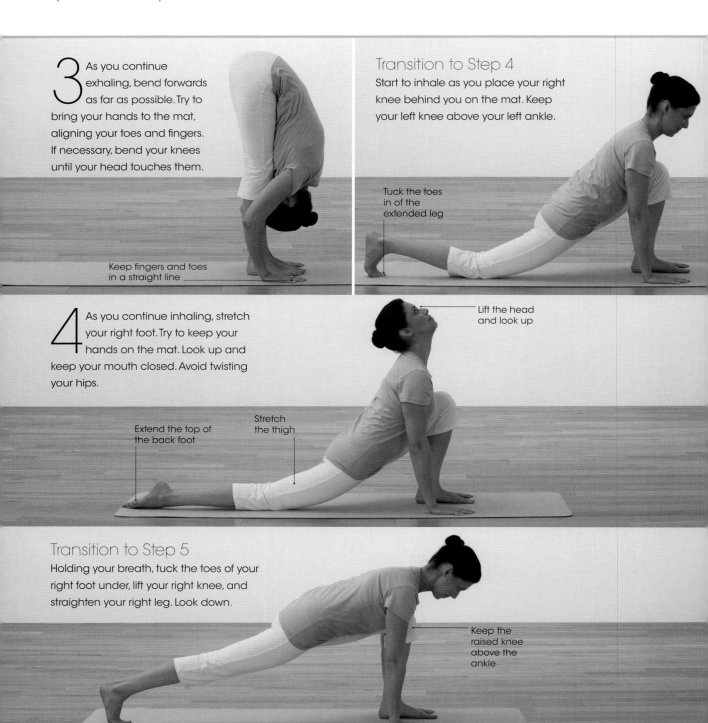

3 As you continue exhaling, bend forwards as far as possible. Try to bring your hands to the mat, aligning your toes and fingers. If necessary, bend your knees until your head touches them.

Keep fingers and toes in a straight line

Transition to Step 4
Start to inhale as you place your right knee behind you on the mat. Keep your left knee above your left ankle.

Tuck the toes in of the extended leg

Lift the head and look up

4 As you continue inhaling, stretch your right foot. Try to keep your hands on the mat. Look up and keep your mouth closed. Avoid twisting your hips.

Extend the top of the back foot

Stretch the thigh

Transition to Step 5
Holding your breath, tuck the toes of your right foot under, lift your right knee, and straighten your right leg. Look down.

Keep the raised knee above the ankle

5 Continuing to hold your breath, take your left leg beside your right leg. Align your head, back, hips, and legs. Straighten the legs and look down towards the floor.

Keep the body straight

Transition to Step 6
Start to exhale as you lower your knees to the mat.

Hands remain in position

6 Continuing to exhale, lower your chest and align your shoulders with your fingertips. Take your forehead to the mat, keeping your hips raised.

Keep the hips raised

Place the forehead on the floor

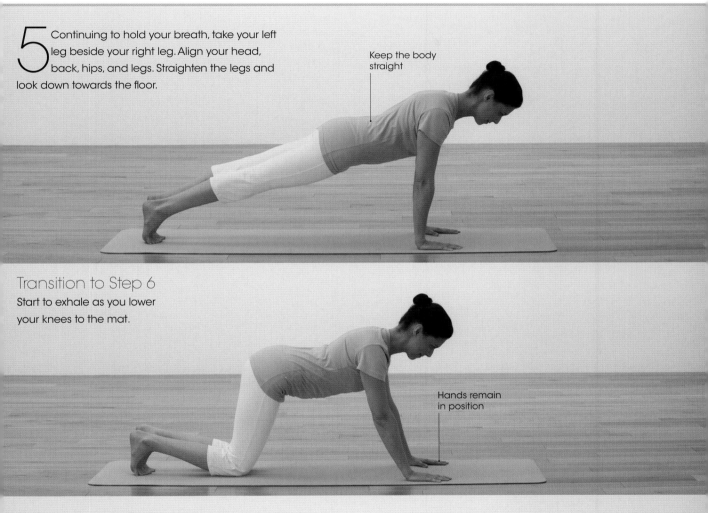

Sun Salutation
(continued)

Transition (a) to Step 7

Start to inhale and, keeping your chest, hands, and forehead in position, lower your hips to the mat. Stretch out your legs and feet.

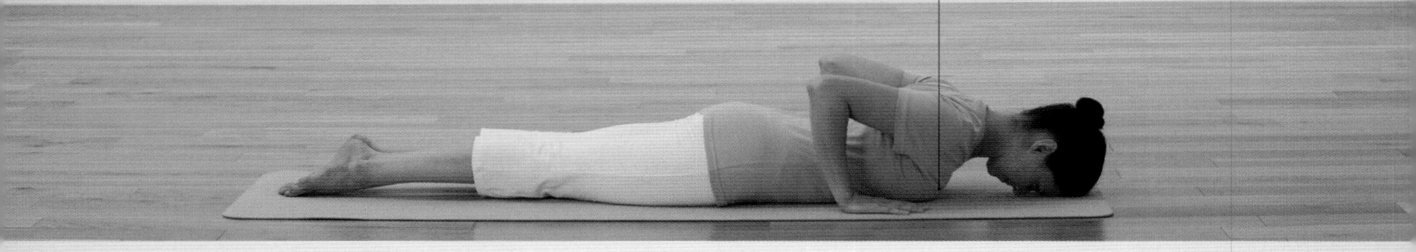

Head and chest start sliding forwards

Transition (b) to Step 7

As you continue inhaling, lift your head and shoulders. Keep your chest on the floor, elbows close to your body, and shoulder blades pulled together. Look up.

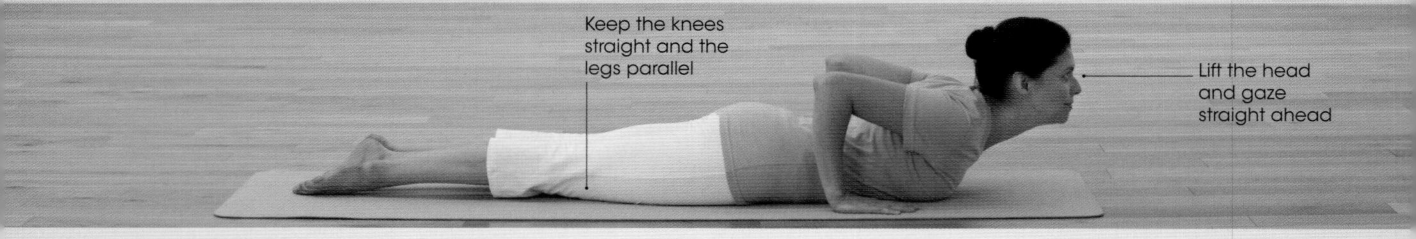

Keep the knees straight and the legs parallel

Lift the head and gaze straight ahead

7 Continue inhaling, arch your head and upper spine backwards, keeping your hips on the mat and your shoulders away from your ears. Look up.

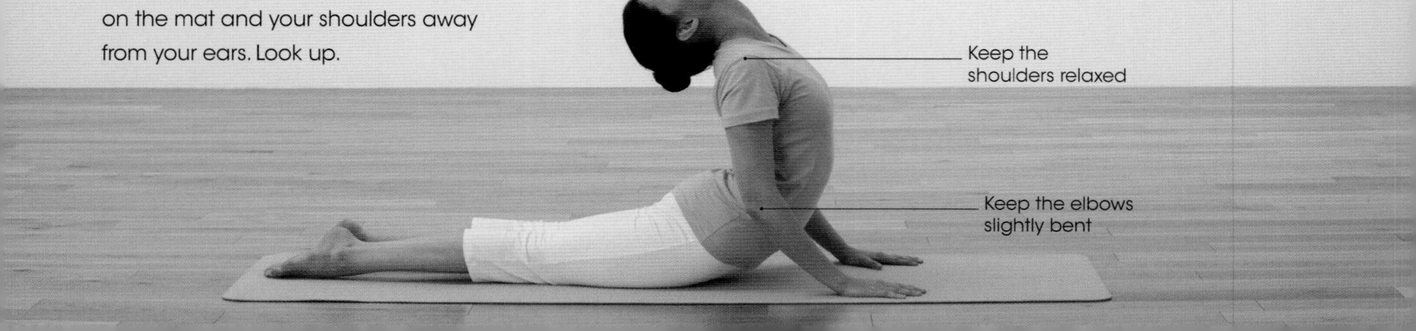

Keep the shoulders relaxed

Keep the elbows slightly bent

Transition to Step 8

Start to exhale as you release your neck and upper back. Tuck your toes under, straighten your legs, and lift your knees off the floor.

Tuck the toes under

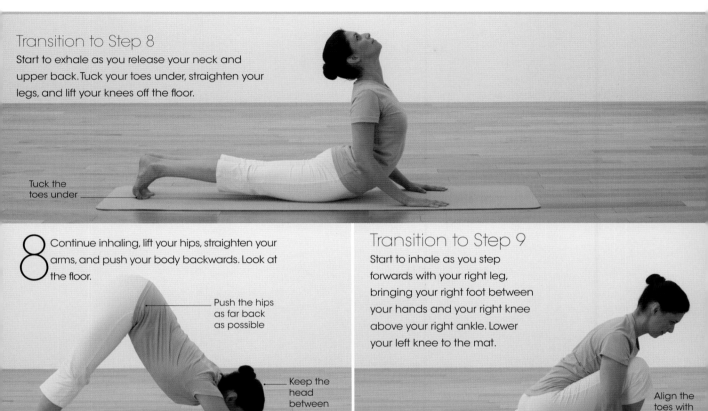

8 Continue inhaling, lift your hips, straighten your arms, and push your body backwards. Look at the floor.

Push the hips as far back as possible

Keep the head between the arms

Transition to Step 9

Start to inhale as you step forwards with your right leg, bringing your right foot between your hands and your right knee above your right ankle. Lower your left knee to the mat.

Align the toes with the fingertips

9 As you continue inhaling, stretch your left foot backwards. Try to keep your hands flat on the mat. Look up and extend your neck and upper back. Keep your hips level. Keep your mouth closed.

Keep the back knee on the floor

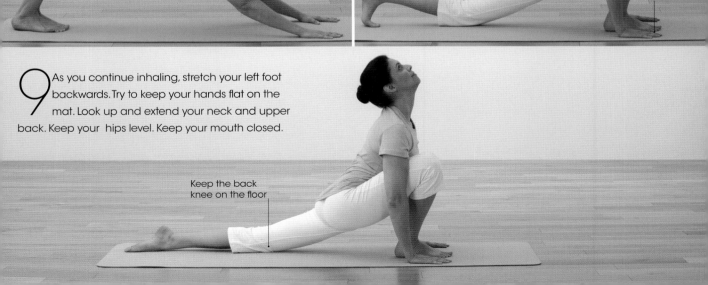

Sun Salutation
(continued)

Transition to Step 10

Start to exhale as you bring your left leg forwards to meet the right, aligning your toes and fingertips and keeping your knees straight. Bend forwards from the waist, but try not to bend your upper back. Look to the floor in front of you.

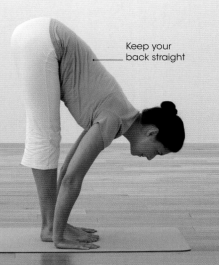

Keep your back straight

10
As you continue exhaling, bend forwards as much as possible, stretching the muscles of your legs and lower back. If necessary, bend your knees until you can touch them with your head.

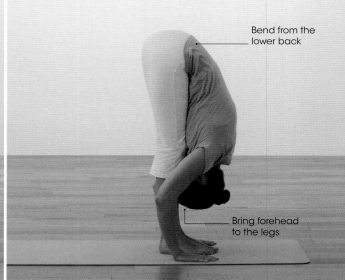

Bend from the lower back

Bring forehead to the legs

Transition (a) to Step 11

Start to inhale as you lift your spine forwards from your waist, keeping your legs straight. Take your arms to your ears. Use the muscles of your back, shoulders, and neck to bring your spine, head, and arms into a horizontal line.

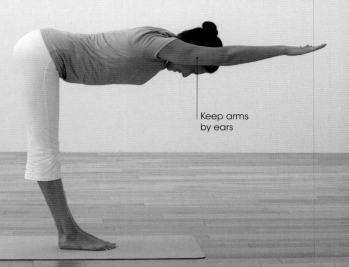

Keep arms by ears

Transition (b) to Step 11

Continuing to inhale, stretch your arms up to your ears, palms facing forwards. As you lift your shoulders, avoid any tension in the neck.

Keep the head, neck, and back in alignment

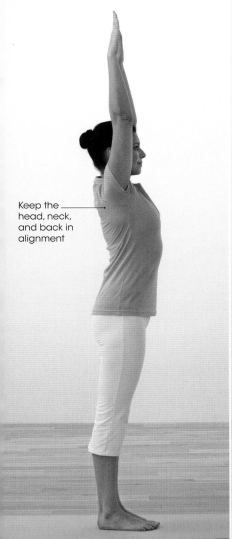

11 Still continuing to inhale, take your weight onto your heels and look upwards as you arch your arms, head, and chest backwards. Stretch the muscles of your chest and abdomen.

Keep elbows straight

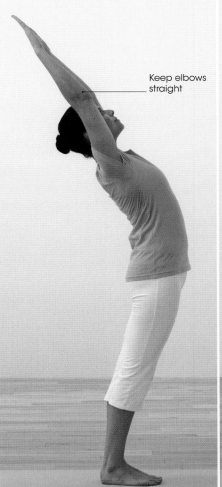

12 Exhale as you lower your arms next to your body. Keep your spine upright and look straight ahead. Take a long inhalation, then continue with a second Sun Salutation, starting at Step 1. This time take your left knee to the mat in Step 4 and your right knee to the mat in Step 9.

Keep arms and hands relaxed

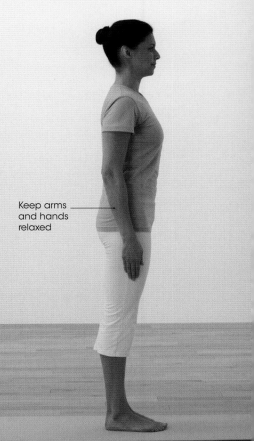

Single Leg Lifts
All Levels

Single Leg Lifts improve the flexibility of the hamstring and calf muscles, which in turn helps prepare for the stretching of the back muscles in the various forward-bending asanas.

Single Leg Lift
Beginner

1 Lie flat on your back with your legs together, arms next to your body, and palms face down.

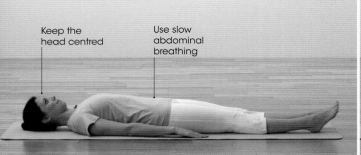

Keep the head centred

Use slow abdominal breathing

2 Inhale and raise your left leg, keeping your knee straight, toes towards your head. Exhale and lower your leg to the starting position. Repeat up to 5 times on each side, then continue with Head to Knee Raise or Deep Stretch Single Leg Lift.

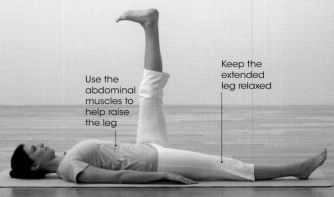

Use the abdominal muscles to help raise the leg

Keep the extended leg relaxed

Head to Knee Raise
Beginner

1 Starting from Single Leg Lift Step 2 (see above), with an exhalation, bend your left leg, and clasp your hands around your left knee, pushing your left thigh firmly against your abdomen.

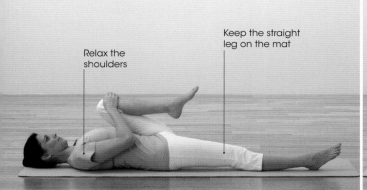

Relax the shoulders

Keep the straight leg on the mat

2 With an inhalation, lift your head and try to bring your forehead against your left knee. With an exhalation, lower your head, arms, and leg. Repeat on the opposite side. Practise up to three Head to Knee Raises on each side.

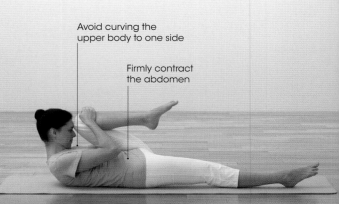

Avoid curving the upper body to one side

Firmly contract the abdomen

Deep Stretch Single Leg Lift
Intermediate

1 Starting from Single Leg Lift Step 2 (see opposite), with an exhalation, take hold of your left leg or foot with both hands, lift your back off the mat, and try to bring your chest and head close to the raised leg.

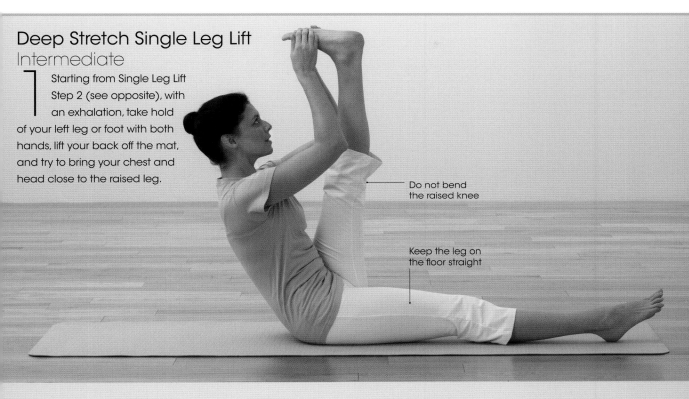

Do not bend
the raised knee

Keep the leg on
the floor straight

2 Inhale and lower your head and back to the mat as you take your left leg over your head. Then exhale and lower your leg and arms back to the starting position. To increase the stretch further, hold for up to one minute as you practise rhythmical abdominal breathing, then release with an exhalation. Repeat on the other side.

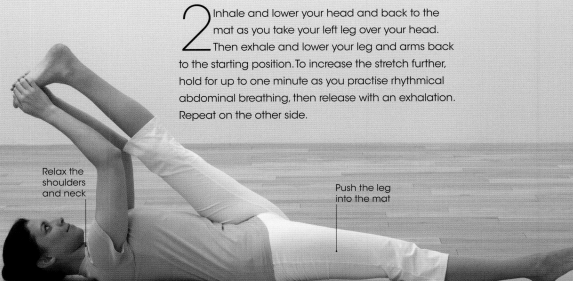

Relax the
shoulders
and neck

Push the leg
into the mat

Double Leg Lifts
Intermediate and Advanced

These Double Leg Lifts provide abdominal strength, which is needed for many asanas, such as Headstand (see pp62–71). After doing Single then Double Leg Lifts, relax in Corpse Pose (see p188).

Arms by Sides
Intermediate

1 Lie flat on your back with your legs together, arms next to your body, and palms face down. Breathe slowly and rhythmically.

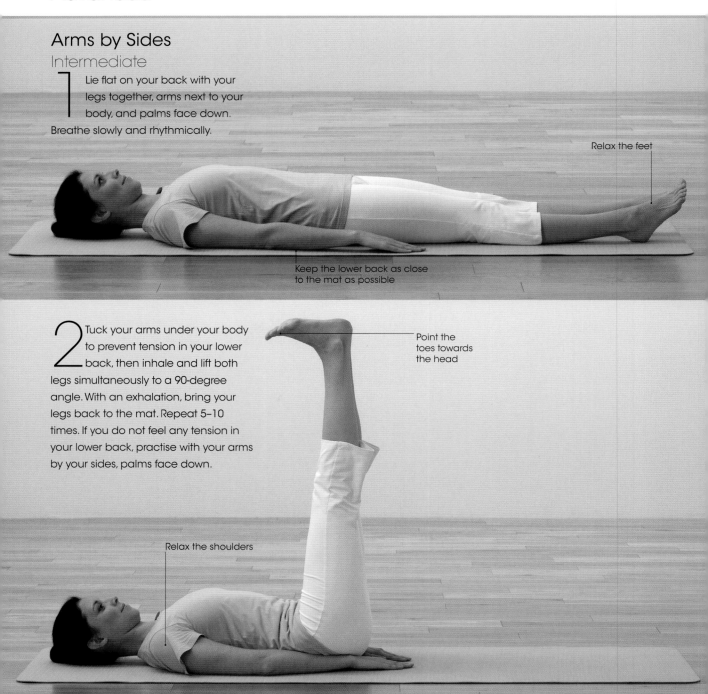

Relax the feet

Keep the lower back as close to the mat as possible

2 Tuck your arms under your body to prevent tension in your lower back, then inhale and lift both legs simultaneously to a 90-degree angle. With an exhalation, bring your legs back to the mat. Repeat 5–10 times. If you do not feel any tension in your lower back, practise with your arms by your sides, palms face down.

Point the toes towards the head

Relax the shoulders

Arms Overhead
Advanced

1 Lie flat on your back, extend your arms on the floor behind you, and catch hold of your elbows. Breathe slowly and rhythmically.

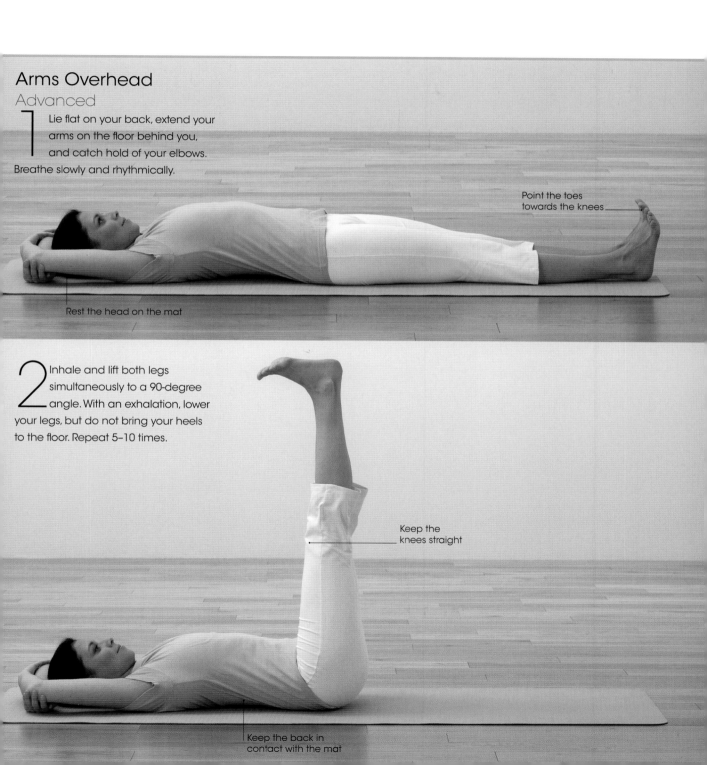

Point the toes towards the knees

Rest the head on the mat

2 Inhale and lift both legs simultaneously to a 90-degree angle. With an exhalation, lower your legs, but do not bring your heels to the floor. Repeat 5–10 times.

Keep the knees straight

Keep the back in contact with the mat

1 Headstand
Sirshasana

Known as "King of Asanas", Headstand is a powerful pose for both body and mind. Balance in Headstand requires coordination of the impulses received in the brain from the inner ear, the skin of the arms and hands, the eyes, and various muscles and joints. Relax afterwards in the counterpose, Child's Pose (see p191).

BENEFITS

PHYSICAL
- Creates a stronger heartbeat.
- Relieves varicose veins.
- Reduces pressure in the lower back.
- Helps to build muscle strength in the shoulder girdle.
- Improves coordination of the body's voluntary and involuntary functions.

MENTAL
- Improves memory and concentration.
- Improves body–mind coordination.
- Enhances intellectual capacities.

CAUTION Do not practise Headstand: if you suffer from high blood pressure; during menstruation; if you suffer from eye conditions such as detached retina or glaucoma; if you have any inflammation in the head area; if you suffer from neck pain due to an accident or other causes. If in doubt, consult your doctor.

Dolphin
Preparatory Exercise for All Levels

1 This exercise prepares you physically and mentally for Headstand. From a kneeling position, lean forwards and place your arms about 20cm (8in) away from your knees on the floor in front of you. Firmly interlock your fingers and close your palms.

2 Without moving your feet away from your arms, inhale and raise your hips.

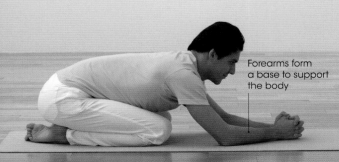

Forearms form a base to support the body

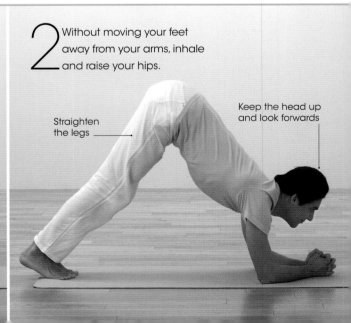

Straighten the legs

Keep the head up and look forwards

3 With an exhalation, rock your whole body forwards and take your head and shoulders down towards the floor. Your hips will now be lower, too.

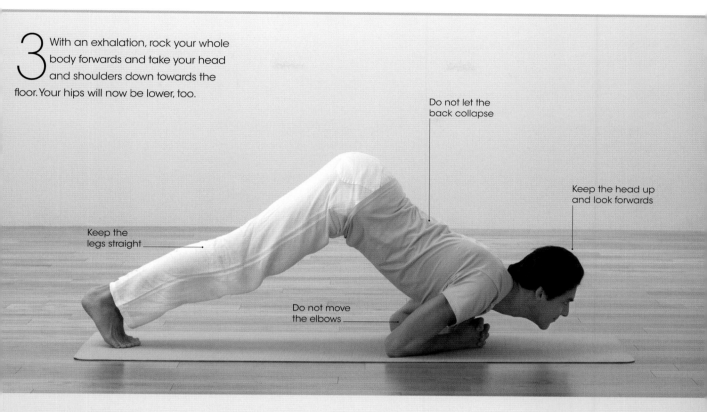

Do not let the back collapse

Keep the head up and look forwards

Keep the legs straight

Do not move the elbows

4 Inhale and push your head and shoulders back up. Your hips will come back up, too. Repeat Steps 1–4 a total of 5–10 times, then bend your knees to the floor.

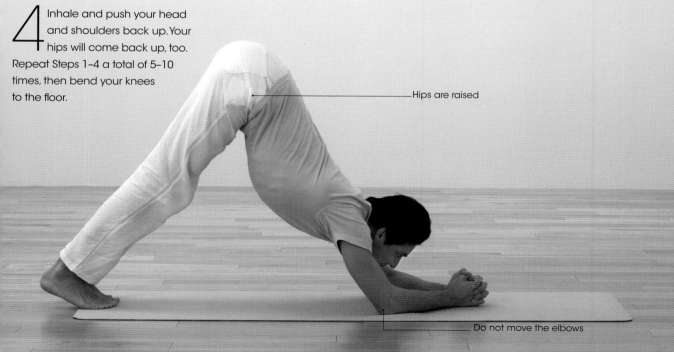

Hips are raised

Do not move the elbows

Headstand
Beginner

Think: "my arms are my legs". These are the instructions that Swami Vishnudevananda used to help students to focus on the tripod base formed by their elbows and hands in this pose.

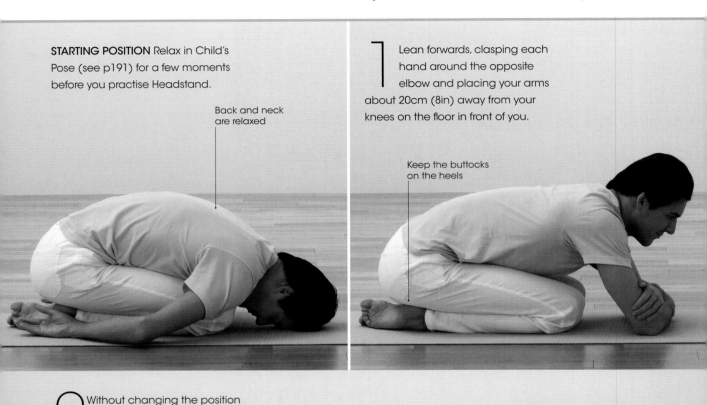

STARTING POSITION Relax in Child's Pose (see p191) for a few moments before you practise Headstand.

Back and neck are relaxed

1 Lean forwards, clasping each hand around the opposite elbow and placing your arms about 20cm (8in) away from your knees on the floor in front of you.

Keep the buttocks on the heels

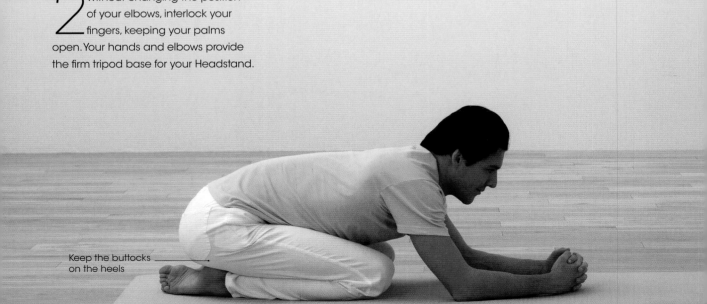

2 Without changing the position of your elbows, interlock your fingers, keeping your palms open. Your hands and elbows provide the firm tripod base for your Headstand.

Keep the buttocks on the heels

3 Bend over and place the topmost part of your head on the floor, firmly pressing the tripod of elbows and hands against the mat.

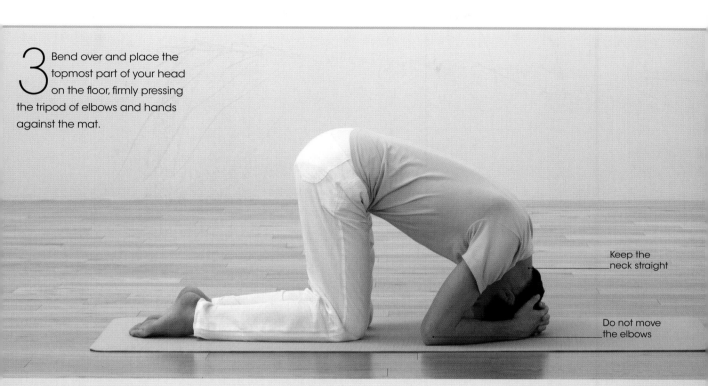

Keep the neck straight

Do not move the elbows

4 Lift your knees off the mat and push your hips up. Hold for a few rhythmical breaths, then return to Child's Pose (see opposite, above left). If you are stiff in the legs or if your elbows start to lift off the floor, do not continue with Step 5, but instead practise Dolphin again (see pp62–3) and Single Leg Lift (see p58).

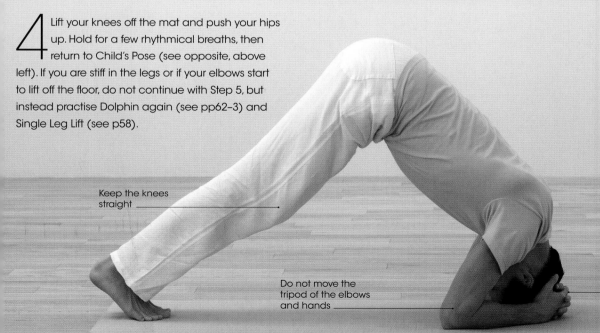

Keep the knees straight

Do not move the tripod of the elbows and hands

Press the forearms and hands against the floor

Headstand
Intermediate and Advanced

You should not practise Headstand against a wall. The secret of success in this pose is to focus on the tripod base formed by your elbows and hands, and on the point of balance in your lower back.

Start with

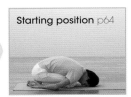 Starting position p64

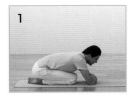 1

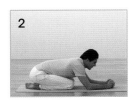 2

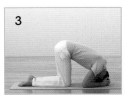 3

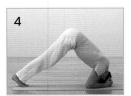 4

5 Starting from Headstand Step 4, and keeping your legs straight, walk your toes as close to your head as possible. Do not allow your back to collapse.

6 Breathing slowly and rhythmically, bend your legs and use your lower back muscles to pull your legs and pelvis up, until you are firmly balanced on your tripod base. Occasional contraction of your abdominal muscles will prevent you from falling over.

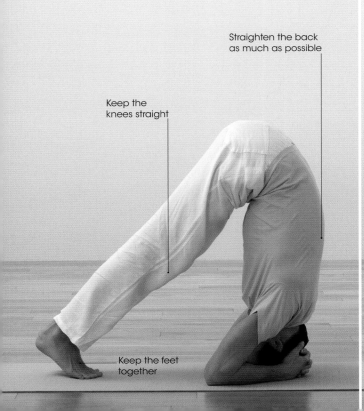

Straighten the back as much as possible

Keep the knees straight

Keep the feet together

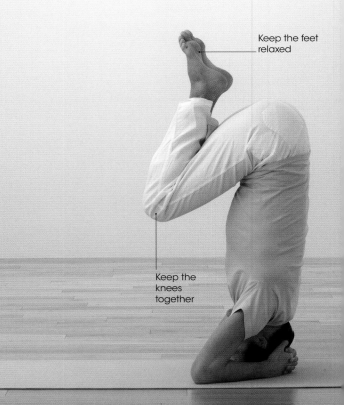

Keep the feet relaxed

Keep the knees together

"Sirshasana [Headstand] invigorates, energises, and vivifies. It is a true blessing and a nectar. You will find real pleasure and exhilaration of spirit in this asana."

Swami Sivananda

7 Continue to breathe rhythmically. Firmly press the tripod of elbows and hands against the floor. Focus on the point of balance in your lower back, then slowly start lifting your knees until your thighs are vertical and your feet are behind you.

8 To come into the full pose, extend your knees and take your legs straight up. Avoid any tension in your legs and feet. Hold for 1–5 minutes, then come down by following Steps 7–1, in that order. Relax in Child's Pose (see p191) for at least 6 deep breaths, then lie in Corpse Pose (see p188) for 1 minute.

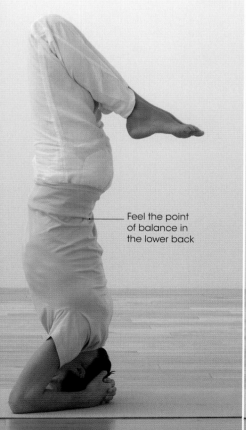

Feel the point of balance in the lower back

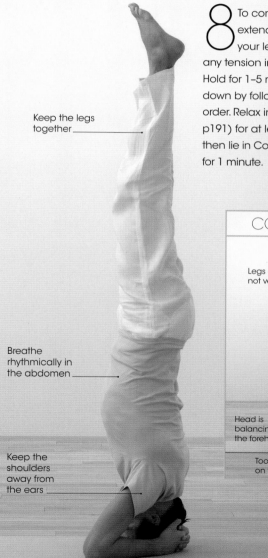

Keep the legs together

Breathe rhythmically in the abdomen

Keep the shoulders away from the ears

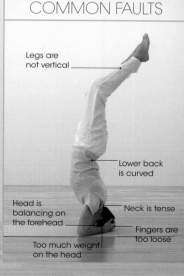

COMMON FAULTS

Legs are not vertical

Lower back is curved

Head is balancing on the forehead

Neck is tense

Fingers are too loose

Too much weight on the head

Headstand
Variations

Each of these Headstand variations helps you to improve your balance, coordination, and powers of concentration. Move carefully until, in the end, your legs move as freely as if they were arms.

Start with

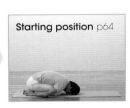

Starting position p64

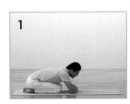

1

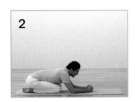

2

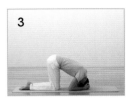

3

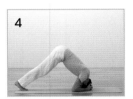

4

Legs to the Sides
Advanced

Starting from Headstand Step 8, with an exhalation, open your legs to the sides and let gravity pull them down towards the floor. Hold for up to 1 minute with deep, rhythmical breathing.

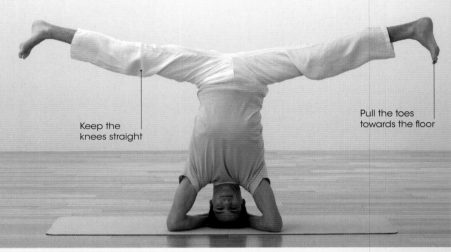

Keep the knees straight

Pull the toes towards the floor

Legs to Front and Back
Advanced

Starting from Headstand Step 8, with an exhalation, slowly take one leg forwards and the other leg equally far back. Change legs. If your Headstand is well balanced, you can alternate your legs in a flowing rhythm, with deep, rhythmical breathing for up to 1 minute.

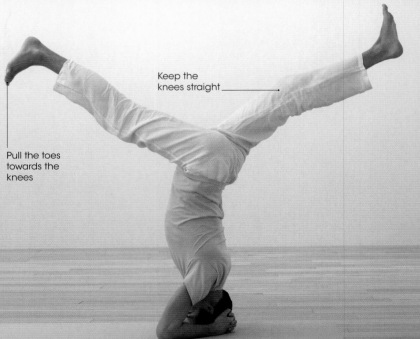

Keep the knees straight

Pull the toes towards the knees

After each variation, bring your legs back together into Headstand Step 8, then either practise another variation or come down by doing Steps 7–1 in that order. Relax afterwards in Child's Pose (see p191).

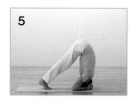

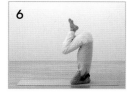

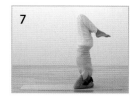

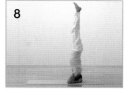

Knees Bent to the Sides
Advanced

Starting from Headstand Step 8, with an exhalation, bend your knees to the sides and carefully bring the soles of your feet together. Hold for up to 1 minute with deep, rhythmical breathing.

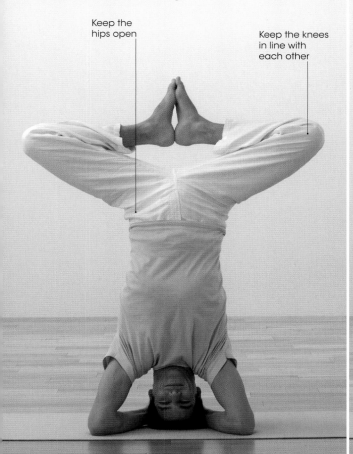

Keep the hips open

Keep the knees in line with each other

One Leg to the Ground
Advanced

Starting from Headstand Step 8, with an exhalation, lower your right leg towards the ground as far as you can. Inhale and raise the leg up again. Repeat on the opposite side. Continue, alternating sides, for up to 1 minute with deep, rhythmical breathing.

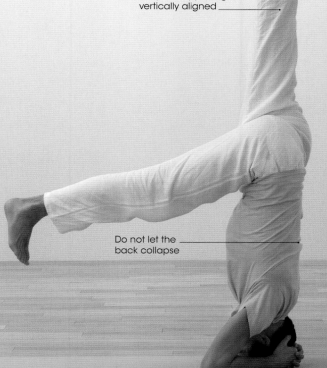

Keep the upper leg vertically aligned

Do not let the back collapse

Headstand
Variations (continued)

These advanced variations teach you to bend and twist in Headstand. Movements of the spine like these give your back an excellent workout – even while you are on your head.

Start with

| Starting position p64 | 1 | 2 | 3 | 4 |

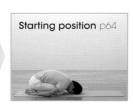 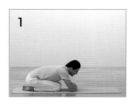 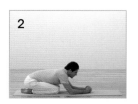 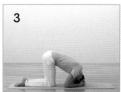 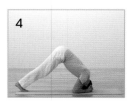

Both Legs to the Ground
Advanced

Starting from Headstand Step 8, with an exhalation and keeping your legs together, lower them in a controlled manner as far as possible towards the floor. With the next inhalation, bring the legs back up. Repeat the movement up to 5 times.

Lotus Headstand
Advanced

Starting from Headstand Step 8, with an exhalation, bring your legs into Lotus (see p114). Hold for up to 1 minute, breathing rhythmically, then uncross your legs, cross them the other way, and hold for up to 1 minute more.

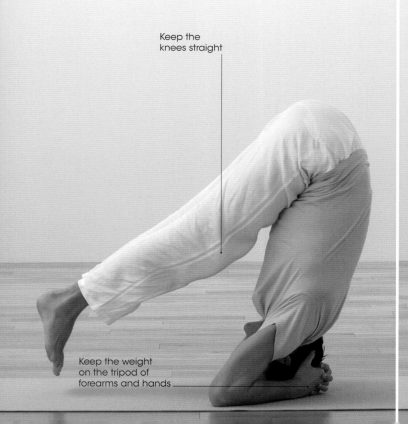

Keep the knees straight

Keep the weight on the tripod of forearms and hands

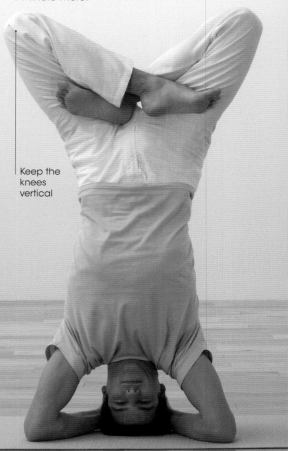

Keep the knees vertical

After each variation, bring your legs back together into Headstand Step 8, then either practise another variation, or come down by doing Steps 7–1 in that order. Relax afterwards in Child's Pose (see p191).

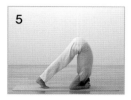
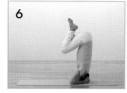
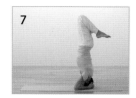
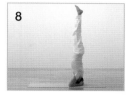

Twisted Lotus Headstand
Advanced
Starting from Lotus Headstand (see opposite), with an exhalation, twist your spine to one side. After a few breaths, slowly twist to the other side. Undo your legs, cross them the other way, and repeat.

To help you balance, concentrate on the tripod of elbows and hands

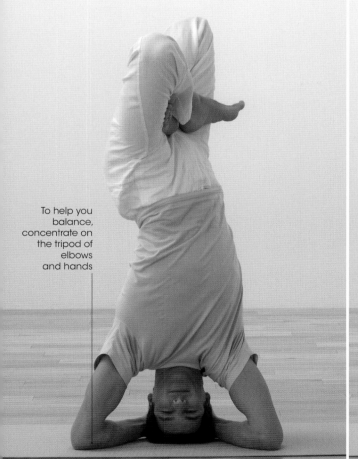

Forward Bend Lotus Headstand
Advanced
Starting from Lotus Headstand (see opposite), with an exhalation, start bending forwards from the hips. Hold for 3 breaths, with each exhalation trying to bend a little lower. Inhale and come back up into Lotus Headstand. Repeat twice more.

Keep the hips lifted

Open the chest

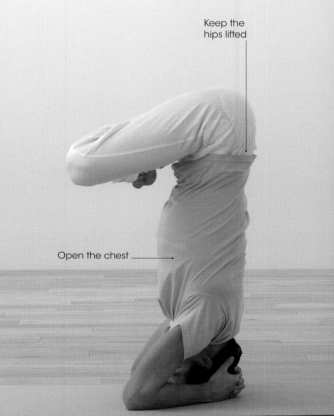

Scorpion
Advanced

Once you feel secure in Headstand and can hold it for at least 2 minutes, you can attempt Scorpion. Get used to arching your body backwards. You will soon be balancing in Scorpion.

Start with

Starting position p64	1	2	3	4

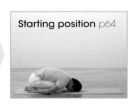 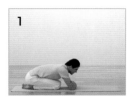 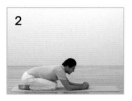 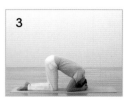 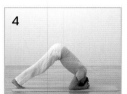

9 Starting from Headstand Step 8, press down on the tripod base formed by your elbows and hands. With an exhalation, bend your body backwards as you push your hips forwards.

10 Staying firm in your forearms and shoulders, and breathing deeply and rhythmically, separate your hands to about shoulder-width apart. Place your palms flat on the floor either side of your head.

11 To come into the full pose, with an inhalation, lift your head and find your balance on your forearms. Hold the pose for up to 30 seconds.

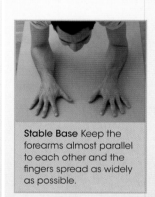

Stable Base Keep the forearms almost parallel to each other and the fingers spread as widely as possible.

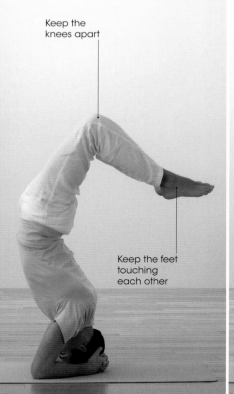

Keep the knees apart

Keep the feet touching each other

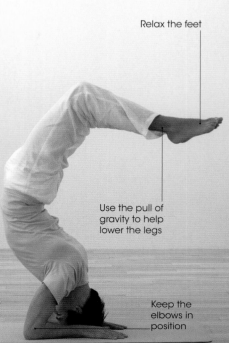

Relax the feet

Use the pull of gravity to help lower the legs

Keep the elbows in position

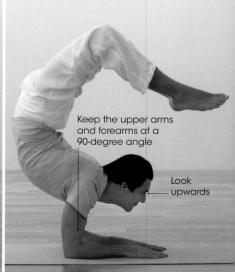

Keep the upper arms and forearms at a 90-degree angle

Look upwards

After practising Scorpion or its variations, return to Headstand Step 8, then either practise another variation, or come down by doing Steps 7–1 in that order. Relax afterwards in Child's Pose (see p191).

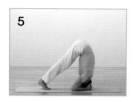

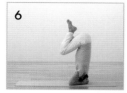

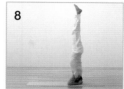

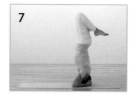

Straight Legs
Variation

Starting from Scorpion Step 11 (see opposite), with an inhalation, straighten your legs. The more you move your legs forwards over your head, the more you have to direct your head and eyes upwards. Hold for up to 30 seconds.

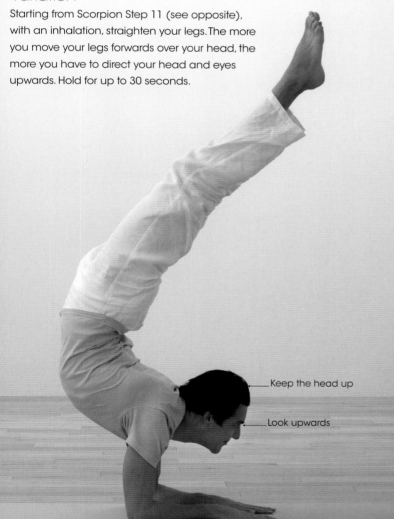

Keep the head up

Look upwards

Feet to Head
Variation

Starting from Scorpion Step 11 (see opposite), with a series of strong exhalations, bend your spine and legs until your feet touch your head. Keep your knees apart to reduce the pressure on your lower back. Hold for up to 30 seconds.

Keep the knees apart

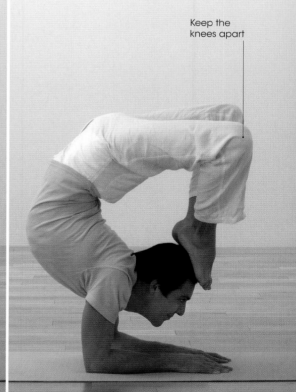

Handstand
Advanced

Handstand offers all the benefits of Headstand. Practise it against a wall until you are confident enough to balance on your hands and arms. Relax afterwards in Child's Pose (see p191).

1 Step one foot in front of the other, then bend forwards and place both hands firmly on the mat, about shoulder-width apart. Keep your back straight and make sure that you do not allow your head to drop.

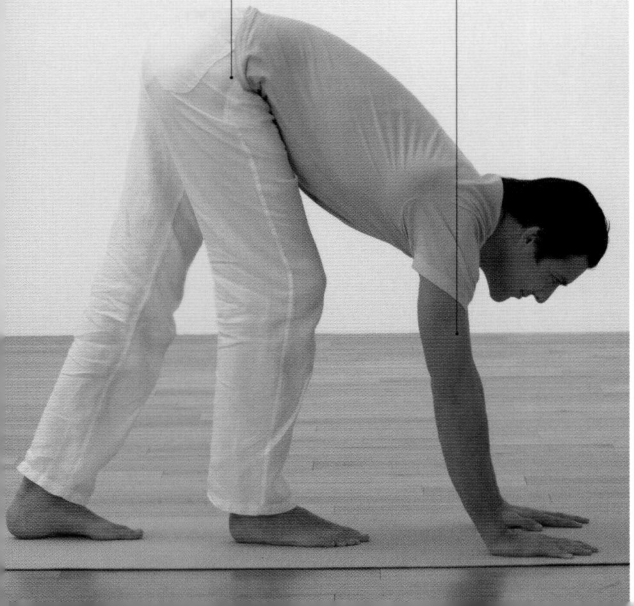

2 On an exhalation, swing your left leg up, followed by your right leg. This involves a pulling motion on your upper leg as you swing it up, and a pushing motion on your lower leg as you jump into position. Stay firm in your arms and hands.

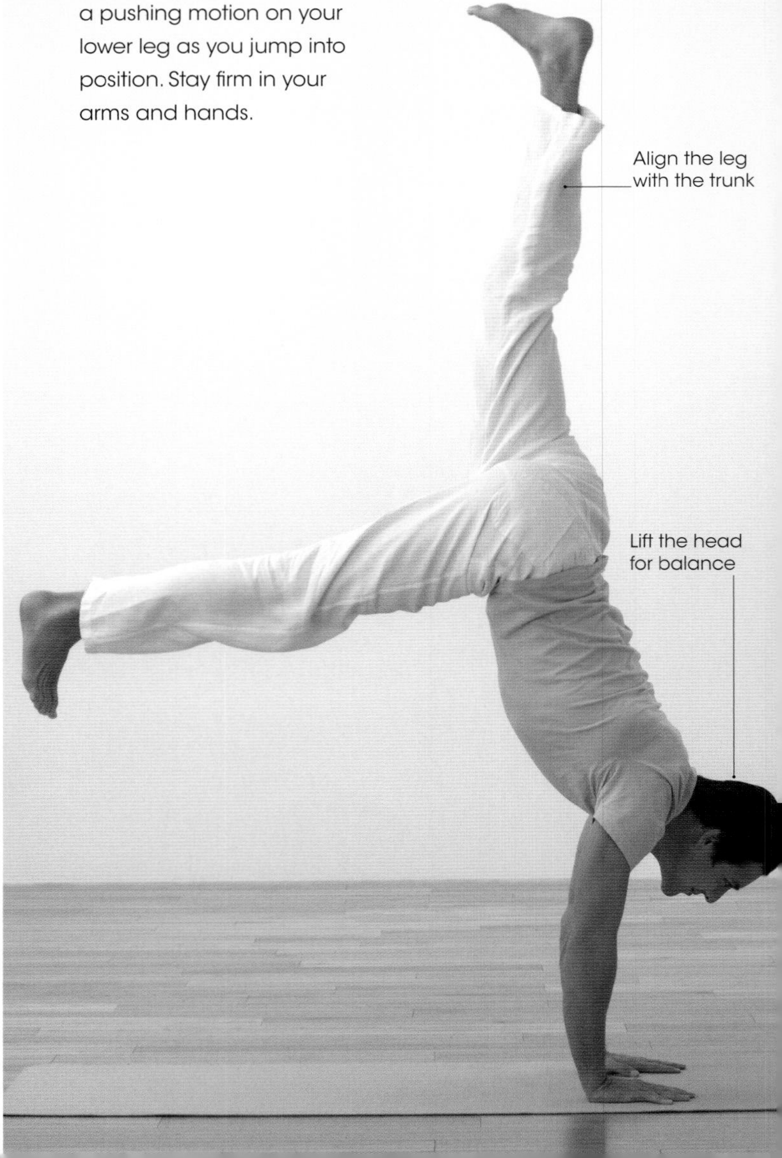

Align the leg with the trunk

Hips are high

Keep the arms straight

Lift the head for balance

3 Keep both legs together as you balance in the full pose. Hold the pose for a few breaths, then come down by bringing one leg at a time to the floor.

Keep the knees straight

Bend the back as little as possible

Scorpion Handstand
Variation

Starting from Handstand Step 3 (see left), bend your spine and legs to bring your feet towards your head. If you are very flexible, you should be able to touch your head with your feet. Come out of the pose by raising your feet back into Handstand, then bringing one leg at a time down to the floor.

Separate the legs

Relax the legs to allow gravity to pull them down

Lift the head as high as possible

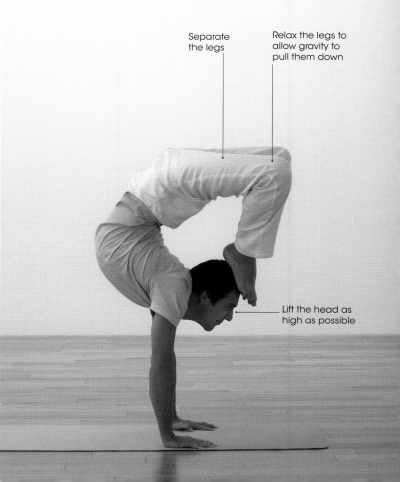

2 Shoulderstand
Sarvangasana

The pressure of the chin against the chest and the inversion of the body in Shoulderstand create the energy flow of Hatha yoga – the union in the solar plexus of the ascending "Ha", or sun, energy with the descending "Tha", or moon, energy. Always practise Fish (see pp92–3) as the counterpose, then relax in Corpse Pose (see p188) for at least 8 breaths.

BENEFITS

PHYSICAL
• Tones and revitalizes the thyroid and parathyroid glands. This improves and balances the metabolism of literally every cell in the body.
• Improves the blood supply to the roots of the spinal nerves.
• Stretches away any stress held in the shoulder and neck area.
• Relieves the pain of varicose veins.

MENTAL
• Stimulates cheerfulness and helps to cure depression.
• Helps to relieve mental sluggishness and promotes clear thinking.

CAUTION If you suffer from high blood pressure, do not hold the pose for more than 30 seconds. If you have a slipped disc or other painful neck condition, practise only as far as Step 3.

Shoulderstand
Beginner

1 Lie flat on your back with your legs together, arms next to your body, and palms touching the mat. Breathe rhythmically in your abdomen.

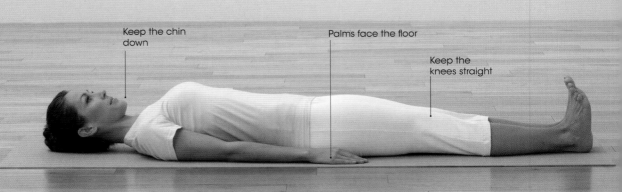

Keep the chin down

Palms face the floor

Keep the knees straight

2 Keeping your back, head, and neck on the mat, inhale and, with your legs straight, lift them to a 90-degree angle.

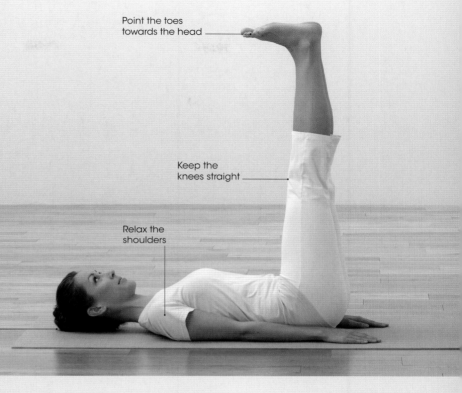

Point the toes towards the head

Keep the knees straight

Relax the shoulders

Keep the head centred

3 On another inhalation, gently lift your legs and hips until you can place your hands and fingers flat against your lower back. Hold for a few rhythmical breaths, then come down by following the instructions on p79.

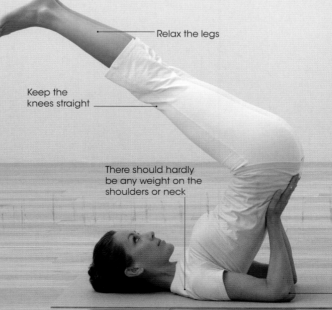

Relax the legs

Keep the knees straight

There should hardly be any weight on the shoulders or neck

Keep the weight on the elbows

Shoulderstand
Intermediate and Advanced

As you progress in Shoulderstand, the more you will be able to align the legs, hips, and back, making it easier to hold the pose, since the back muscles will not need to work so hard against gravity.

Start with

1 p76

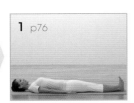

2

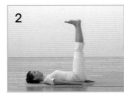

3

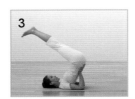

4 To come into the final pose, start from Shoulderstand Step 3. Continue lifting your body until your legs are in a straight line, and bring your chin as close to your chest as possible. Hold for up to 3 minutes.

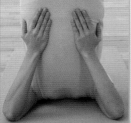

Hand Position Take your hands as close as possible to your shoulder blades, with your arms as parallel to each other as possible.

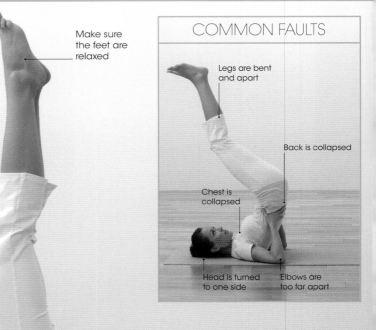

Make sure the feet are relaxed

Breathe rhythmically in the abdomen

Maintain a constant pressure of the hands and arms against the upper back

COMMON FAULTS

Legs are bent and apart

Back is collapsed

Chest is collapsed

Head is turned to one side

Elbows are too far apart

TO COME DOWN, slowly place both arms flat on the floor, palms face down, and bend your hips, bringing both legs slightly behind you, towards the floor. Using your arms as a brake, slowly roll down, vertebra by vertebra. Once your back is flat on the mat, use your abdominal muscles to lower your legs.

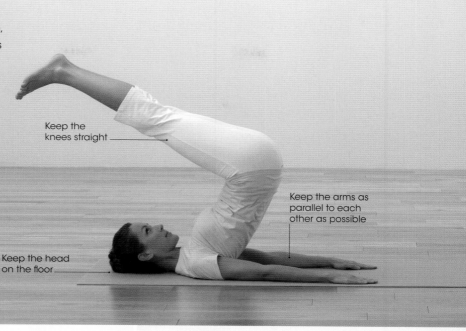

Keep the knees straight

Keep the arms as parallel to each other as possible

Keep the head on the floor

Arms on Floor
Advanced Variation
Starting from Shoulderstand Step 4, slowly place both arms flat on the floor, palms face down. Keep your body upright. Hold for up to 1 minute, then come down by following the instructions above.

Align the legs vertically as much as possible

Push the arms firmly into the mat

Hands on Thighs
Advanced Variation
Starting from Shoulderstand Step 4, slowly lift one arm at a time and take it onto the front of your thigh. Keep your balance on your shoulders, neck, and head. Hold for up to 1 minute, then come down by following the instructions above.

Keep the legs together

Control the balance by breathing rhythmically in the abdomen

3 Plough
Halasana

Plough is a natural continuation of the forward-bending movement that you will have done in Shoulderstand (see pp76–9). The shape you make in this pose, with your feet and hands on the floor, resembles a plough. This asana helps to keep the whole spine youthful. Relax afterwards in Corpse Pose (see p188) for at least 8 breaths.

BENEFITS

PHYSICAL
• Stretches the back of the body completely, which mobilizes the entire spine.
• Loosens tight hamstrings.
• Stretches the deep and superficial muscles of the back.
• Increases the blood supply to the nerves of the spine.
• Releases tension in the shoulder and neck muscles.
• Helps improve the flexibility of the shoulder joint.

• Improves digestion and helps to overcome constipation by placing pressure on the abdominal area.

MENTAL
• By teaching you how to breathe and relax while there is pressure on the front of your body, Plough helps you cope better with any claustrophobia, stress, or sense of being overwhelmed by a lack of space in your daily life.

CAUTION If you are suffering from an acute slipped disc, you should consult your doctor or physiotherapist before starting this exercise.

Plough
Beginner

1 Lie flat on your back with your legs together, arms next to your body, and palms face down on the mat.

Keep the legs together

2 With an inhalation, slowly start lifting both your legs to a 90-degree angle. Keep your arms, head, and shoulders on the floor.

Point the toes towards the head

Keep the knees straight

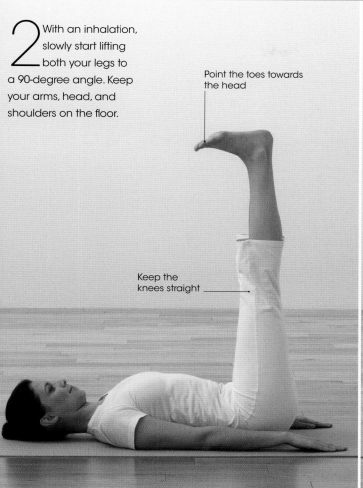

3 With another inhalation, lift your legs and hips until you can place your hands against your lower back.

Keep the toes pointed towards the head

Keep the weight on the elbows

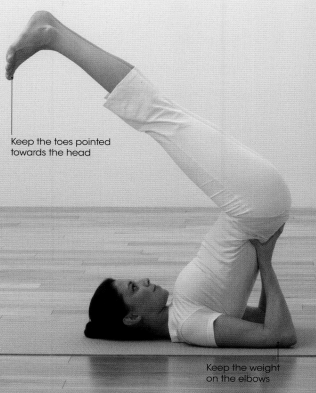

4 With an exhalation, slowly lower your legs behind your head, taking your feet to the floor. If your feet do not reach the floor, hold this pose for 5 breaths, then roll out as described on p83 and relax on your back. Once your feet do reach the floor, continue with Step 5 (see p82).

Make sure the knees are straight

Keep the back supported with the hands

Keep the toes pointing towards the head

Plough
Intermediate and Advanced

At the intermediate level of Plough, you hyperextend your arms as you place them on the floor. This increases your flexibility, not only in your hips and back, but also in your shoulder girdle.

Start with

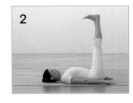

1 p80   2   3   4

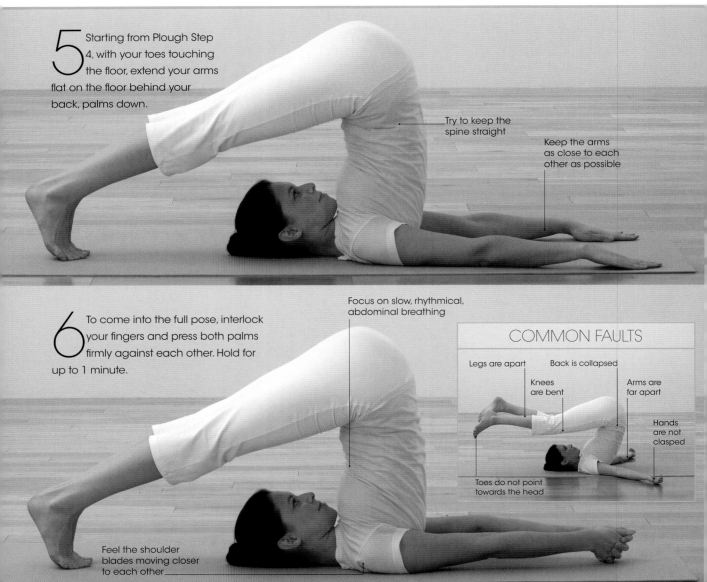

5 Starting from Plough Step 4, with your toes touching the floor, extend your arms flat on the floor behind your back, palms down.

Try to keep the spine straight

Keep the arms as close to each other as possible

6 To come into the full pose, interlock your fingers and press both palms firmly against each other. Hold for up to 1 minute.

Focus on slow, rhythmical, abdominal breathing

Feel the shoulder blades moving closer to each other

COMMON FAULTS

Legs are apart

Back is collapsed

Knees are bent

Arms are far apart

Hands are not clasped

Toes do not point towards the head

*"Never behold life physically.
Understand it psychically,
and realize it spiritually."* Swami Sivananda

TO COME OUT of the pose, release
your hands, place your arms flat on
the floor and raise your legs until they
are parallel to the floor. With an
exhalation, slowly roll down to the floor,
vertebra by vertebra.

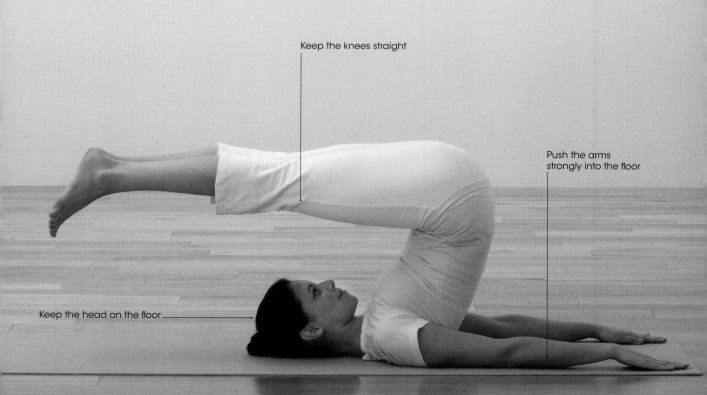

Keep the knees straight

Push the arms
strongly into the floor

Keep the head on the floor

Plough
Variations

As well as working the hips and giving the upper back even more of a stretch, these Plough variations give the solar plexus a powerful massage – as long as you keep up your rhythmical breathing.

Start with

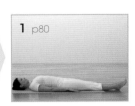

1 p80

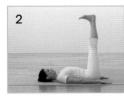

2

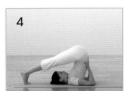

3

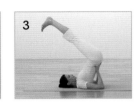

4

Feet Apart
Beginner

Starting from Plough Step 4, take your legs as far apart as possible. Extend your hands flat on the floor behind you, palms face down. Hold for up to 1 minute, then raise your legs until they are parallel to the floor. Come out of the pose as described on p83.

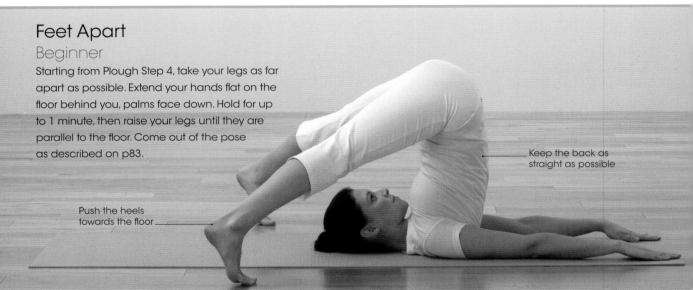

Keep the back as straight as possible

Push the heels towards the floor

Arm Wrap
Intermediate

Starting from Feet Apart (see above), lower your knees next to your ears. Bring your arms over your knees and take your hands to your ears. Hold for up to 1 minute, breathing slowly, then come out of the pose as described on p83.

Stretch the toes

Relax the feet

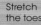

Hands to Feet
Intermediate

Starting from Plough Step 4, take your arms next to your ears and try to touch your toes. Hold for up to 1 minute, breathing slowly. Come out of the pose as described on p83.

Keep the knees straight

"The self-effort of today becomes the destiny of tomorrow. Self-effort and destiny are one and the same." Swami Sivananda

Knees Behind Head
Advanced

Starting from Plough Step 4, walk your feet as far away from your head as possible. Then bend your knees and slowly lower them to the mat behind your head. Hold for up to 30 seconds, then raise your legs until they are parallel to the floor. Come out of the pose as described on p83.

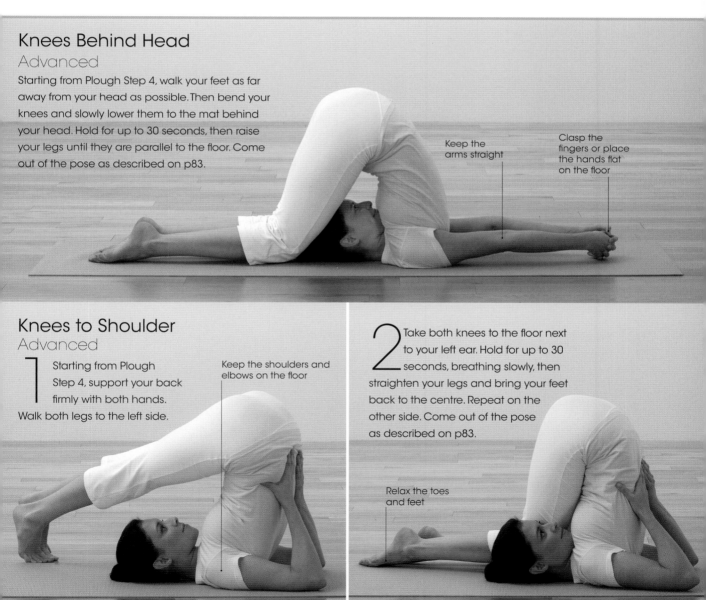

Keep the arms straight

Clasp the fingers or place the hands flat on the floor

Knees to Shoulder
Advanced

1 Starting from Plough Step 4, support your back firmly with both hands. Walk both legs to the left side.

Keep the shoulders and elbows on the floor

2 Take both knees to the floor next to your left ear. Hold for up to 30 seconds, breathing slowly, then straighten your legs and bring your feet back to the centre. Repeat on the other side. Come out of the pose as described on p83.

Relax the toes and feet

Bridge
All Levels

Bridge improves both the flexibility and strength of your spine. Steps 2–4 also provide an excellent training programme for strengthening your wrists. Relax afterwards in Corpse Pose (see p188).

Beginner

1 Lie on your back, with your feet and legs about 50cm (20in) apart, your knees bent, and your feet flat on the floor. Place your arms by your sides, palms face down.

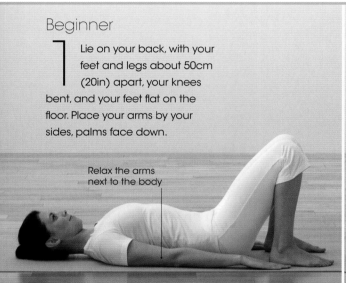

Relax the arms next to the body

2 Catch firmly hold of your ankles, inhale, and push up your hips.

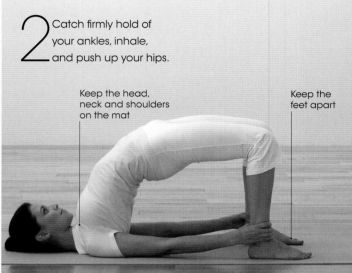

Keep the head, neck and shoulders on the mat

Keep the feet apart

3 Release your hands and place them flat on your back, as close to your shoulder blades as possible. Point your fingers towards your lower back and place your thumbs on your sides. Breathe slowly and deeply. Continue with Step 4 or come out by releasing your hands and lowering your hips.

Place the hands close to the shoulder blades

Keep the feet separate

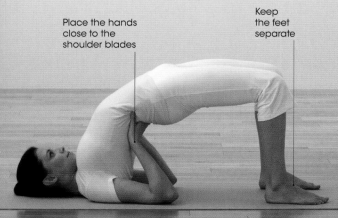

Intermediate

4 Come into the full pose by walking your feet farther away. Hold for up to 30 seconds, breathing deeply. Come out of the pose by walking your feet back towards your body, then release your hands and lower your hips.

COMMON FAULTS

Hands are supporting the waist

Shoulders are not on the mat

Fingers are on the sides of the body

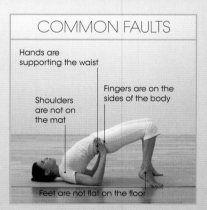

Feet are not flat on the floor

Expand the rib cage

Be strong in the arms and wrists

Keep the legs apart

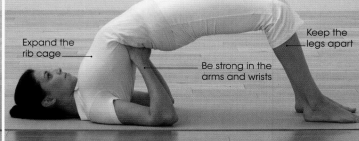

Start with

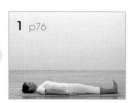
1 p76

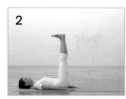
2

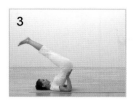
3

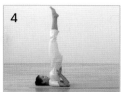
4

Shoulderstand to Bridge
Intermediate Variation

5 Once you have mastered Bridge, try coming into the pose from Shoulderstand Step 4. Push your hands firmly against your back, bend both knees, and keep one leg over your head as you lower the other leg. Then lower the second leg to the floor, keeping your hips up. After a few breaths in Bridge, walk your feet closer to your body and, on an inhalation, lift one leg and then the other back up into Shoulderstand. Come out of the pose as described on p79 and relax.

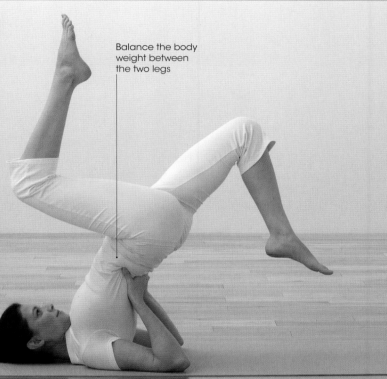

Balance the body weight between the two legs

Shoulderstand to Bridge
Advanced Variation

5 In this advanced starting position, begin with Shoulderstand Step 4, then bend your knees and lower both feet to the floor simultaneously. After a few breaths in Bridge, walk your feet closer to your body and, on an inhalation, lift one leg and then the other back up into Shoulderstand. Come out of the pose as described on p79 and relax.

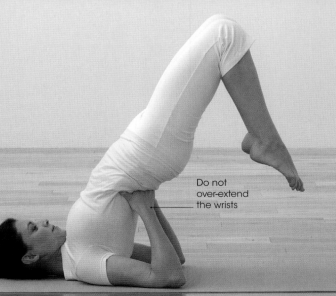

Do not over-extend the wrists

Bridge
Variations

After you have practised these advanced Bridge variations, you should go back into Shoulderstand (see pp76–9) for up to 30 seconds before relaxing in Corpse Pose (see p188).

Start with

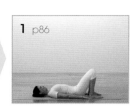

1 p86

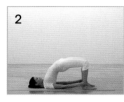

2

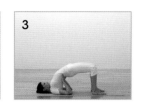

3

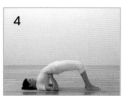

4

Single Leg Lift
Advanced

Starting from Bridge Step 4, lift your left leg straight up as you inhale. After a few deep breaths, lower the leg with an exhalation, then repeat with your right leg. Come out of the pose by releasing your hands and lowering your hips.

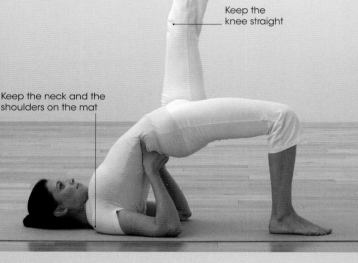

Keep the toes pointed

Keep the knee straight

Keep the neck and the shoulders on the mat

Legs Straight
Advanced

Starting from Bridge Step 4, bring your legs and feet together, then walk your feet away until your legs are completely straight. Hold for up to 30 seconds, breathing deeply. Come out of the pose by walking your feet closer to your body, releasing your hands, and lowering your hips.

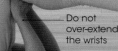

Do not over-extend the wrists

Start with

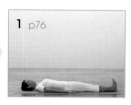

1 p76

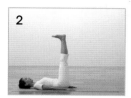

2

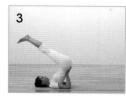

3

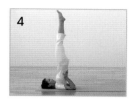

4

Half Lotus Bridge
Advanced

5 Starting from Shoulderstand Step 4, bend your left leg and use your right hand to pull your left foot closer to your hip.

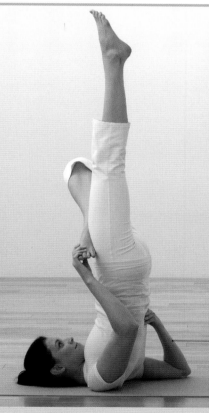

Use the arm to keep your balance

6 Support your back with both hands and slowly bring your right foot down to the floor. Hold for up to 30 seconds, then try to kick back up into Shoulderstand. If you cannot do this, lower your left foot to the floor, release your hands, lower your hips, then inhale and return to Shoulderstand Step 4. Repeat on the opposite side. If you can kick back up into Shoulderstand, come out of the pose as described on p79. Otherwise release your hands and lower your hips.

Bring the knee into a horizontal position

Walk the foot away from the body

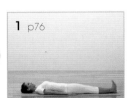

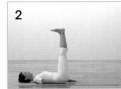

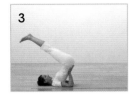

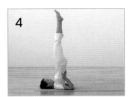

Shoulderstand Cycle
Intermediate

The Shoulderstand Cycle is an excellent exercise for strengthening the muscles of the arms, the back, the abdomen, and the wrists. It also helps you to improve your alignment in Shoulderstand.

Start with

1 p76

2

3

4

5 Starting with Shoulderstand Step 4, position your arms and hands firmly.

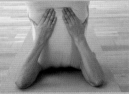

Hand Position Take your hands as close as possible to your shoulder blades, with your arms as parallel to each other as possible.

6 On an exhalation, come into Single Leg Plough by lowering your left leg over your head until your toes reach the floor. Inhale and bring your leg back. Repeat, lowering your right leg.

Keep the upper leg straight and vertical

7 On an exhalation, transition into Plough by lowering both legs over your head until your toes reach the floor.

Keep the spine straight

Keep the back supported with both hands

8 Come back into Shoulderstand by lifting both legs simultaneously on an inhalation. If you find this difficult, you may move your hips forwards slightly, then lift your legs. This lessens the impact of the weight of your legs on your back muscles.

Keep the knees straight

Use your back muscles to lift the legs

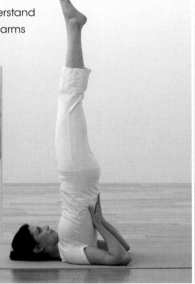

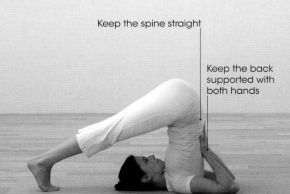

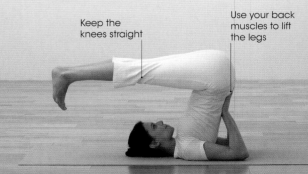

"Health is Wealth.
Peace of Mind is Happiness.
Yoga shows the Way." Swami Vishnudevananda

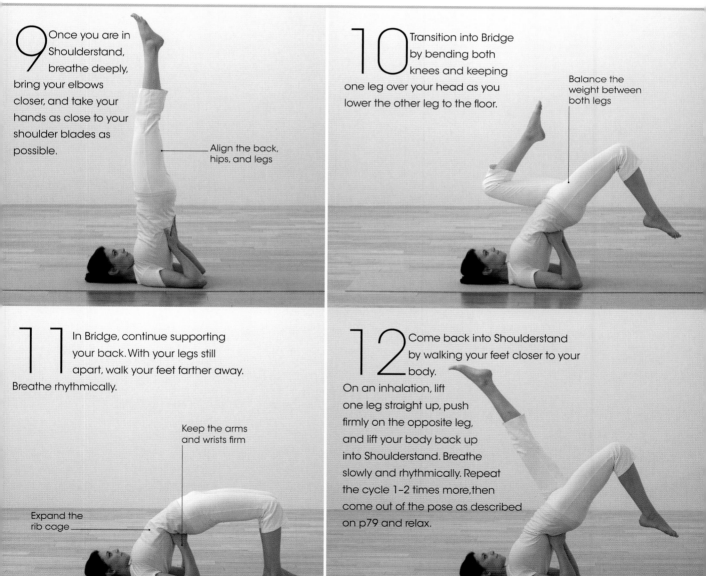

9 Once you are in Shoulderstand, breathe deeply, bring your elbows closer, and take your hands as close to your shoulder blades as possible.

Align the back, hips, and legs

10 Transition into Bridge by bending both knees and keeping one leg over your head as you lower the other leg to the floor.

Balance the weight between both legs

11 In Bridge, continue supporting your back. With your legs still apart, walk your feet farther away. Breathe rhythmically.

Keep the arms and wrists firm

Expand the rib cage

12 Come back into Shoulderstand by walking your feet closer to your body.
On an inhalation, lift one leg straight up, push firmly on the opposite leg, and lift your body back up into Shoulderstand. Breathe slowly and rhythmically. Repeat the cycle 1–2 times more, then come out of the pose as described on p79 and relax.

4 Fish
Matsyasana

Fish bends your spine in the opposite direction to Shoulderstand (see pp76–9) and is the counterpose to the Shoulderstand cycle. Spend at least half as much time doing Fish as you spend doing Shoulderstand. After you have practised Fish, you will find that you experience a much deeper relaxation in the resting position of Corpse Pose (see p188).

BENEFITS

PHYSICAL
• Relieves stiffness in the neck and shoulders.
• Corrects any tendency to round the shoulders.
• Strengthens the arm muscles.
• Expands the rib cage.
• Helps to tone the nerves of the neck and back area.
• Together with Shoulderstand, helps to improve the functioning of the thyroid and parathyroid glands.
• Improves the capacity of the lungs.
• Decongests the lungs.
• Relieves asthma.

MENTAL
• The wide opening of the rib cage reduces the pressure on the abdomen and recharges the solar plexus. This helps to overcome depression.

CAUTION If the hyper-extension of the neck causes any discomfort or dizziness, do not practise the posture or practise it for only a few breaths.

Fish
All Levels

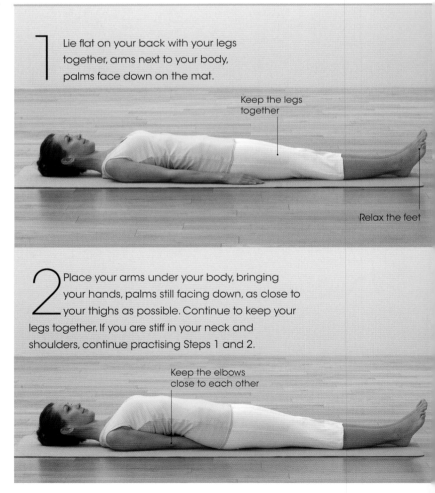

1 Lie flat on your back with your legs together, arms next to your body, palms face down on the mat.

Keep the legs together

Relax the feet

2 Place your arms under your body, bringing your hands, palms still facing down, as close to your thighs as possible. Continue to keep your legs together. If you are stiff in your neck and shoulders, continue practising Steps 1 and 2.

Keep the elbows close to each other

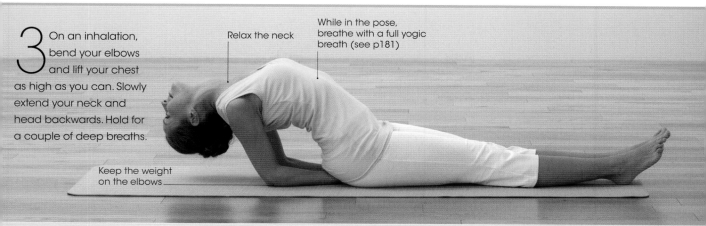

3 On an inhalation, bend your elbows and lift your chest as high as you can. Slowly extend your neck and head backwards. Hold for a couple of deep breaths.

Relax the neck

While in the pose, breathe with a full yogic breath (see p181)

Keep the weight on the elbows

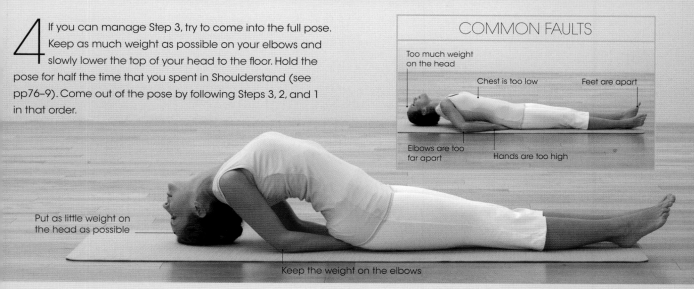

4 If you can manage Step 3, try to come into the full pose. Keep as much weight as possible on your elbows and slowly lower the top of your head to the floor. Hold the pose for half the time that you spent in Shoulderstand (see pp76–9). Come out of the pose by following Steps 3, 2, and 1 in that order.

COMMON FAULTS

Too much weight on the head

Chest is too low

Feet are apart

Elbows are too far apart

Hands are too high

Put as little weight on the head as possible

Keep the weight on the elbows

NECK STRETCH After Fish, practise this pose to release any tension in your neck. With your fingers interlocked behind your head and your forearms close to your ears, inhale and lift your head, pushing your chin into your chest. On an exhalation, slowly lower your head back to the mat. Repeat 2 times. Relax for 1–2 minutes in Corpse Pose (see p188).

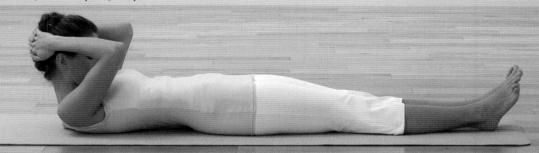

Fish
Variations

Cross-legged Fish adds a deep thigh stretch, while Lotus Fish gives you a stable base, allowing you to intensify the backward bend. End each pose with the Neck stretch (see p93).

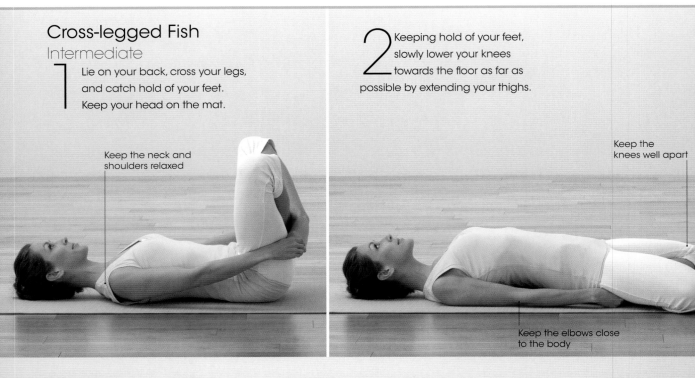

Cross-legged Fish
Intermediate

1 Lie on your back, cross your legs, and catch hold of your feet. Keep your head on the mat.

Keep the neck and shoulders relaxed

2 Keeping hold of your feet, slowly lower your knees towards the floor as far as possible by extending your thighs.

Keep the knees well apart

Keep the elbows close to the body

3 On an inhalation, firmly push on your elbows and move your hips up and forwards, bringing your knees as close to the floor as possible. On another inhalation, lift your chest and bring the top of your head to the floor. Hold for up to 1 minute, then inhale, push your chest higher, and extend your neck. On an exhalation, lower your back to the floor and uncross your legs. Next time you practise this pose, cross your legs the opposite way.

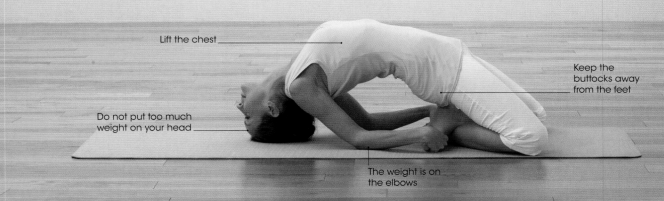

Lift the chest

Keep the buttocks away from the feet

Do not put too much weight on your head

The weight is on the elbows

Start with

1 p114

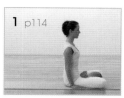

Lotus Fish
Advanced

2 Starting from Lotus final position, slowly lie back on the mat. Place your elbows close to your body and try to catch hold of your toes. Alternatively, place your hands on top of your hips.

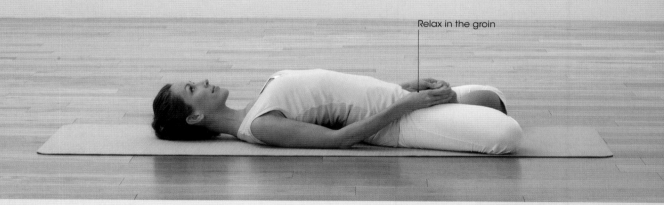

Relax in the groin

3 On an inhalation, bend your elbows and push your chest up. Slowly extend your neck until the top of your head is touching the floor. Hold for up to 1 minute, then inhale, push your chest higher, and extend your neck. On an exhalation, lower your back to the floor and uncross your legs. Next time you practise this pose, position your legs in Lotus in the opposite order.

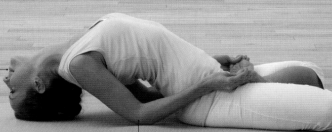

Bring the knees as close to the floor as possible

Keep the mouth closed for maximum stretch of the throat

Keep the elbows firmly on the mat

5 Forward Bend
Paschimotanasana

This pose can be very meditative. If you put equal emphasis on posture, breathing, and relaxation in your practice, this will balance the stimulation provided by the muscle stretches with your body's quiet awareness of the pull of gravity. After Forward Bend, practice Inclined Plane as a counterpose (see p100), then relax in Corpse Pose (see p188).

BENEFITS

PHYSICAL
• Stretches the posterior muscles completely from toes to neck.
• Reduces fat by putting pressure on the abdomen.
• Massages the liver, kidneys, and pancreas.
• Alleviates constipation.
• Relaxes the back muscles.
• Helps control diabetes.
• Calms and soothes the entire nervous system.

MENTAL
• This pose requires conscious control to align toes, knees, and neck correctly, and conscious letting go, by allowing gravity to pull the spine into the pose.
Achieving control with detachment is a benefit that can be applied to daily life, as well as in the practice of meditation.

Forward Bend
Beginner

1 Lie stretched out on your back with your palms face down on your thighs and your legs together. Relax your feet.

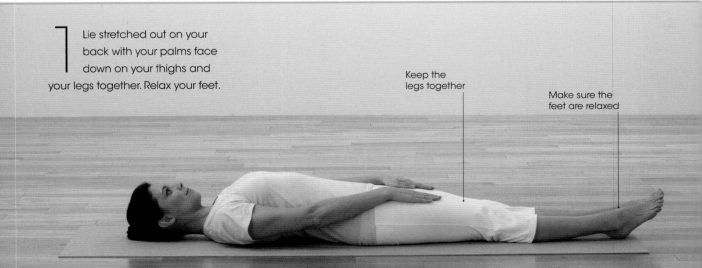

Keep the legs together

Make sure the feet are relaxed

2 On an inhalation, sit up straight with your legs stretched out in front of you. Keep your head, neck, and back in a straight line.

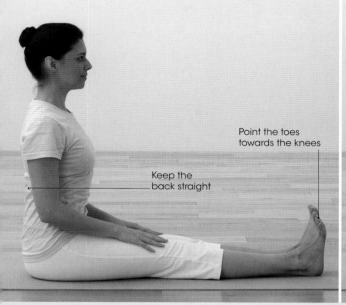

Point the toes towards the knees

Keep the back straight

3 On another inhalation, raise both arms straight up, stretching them as high as possible.

Align the arms with the ears

4 Exhale and bend forwards from the hips. Try to reach your calves or ankles with your hands. Repeat 3–4 times, each time holding the pose for a few breaths more. Continue with Step 5 (see p98) or come back up on an inhalation.

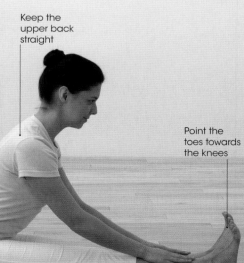

Keep the upper back straight

Point the toes towards the knees

COMMON FAULTS

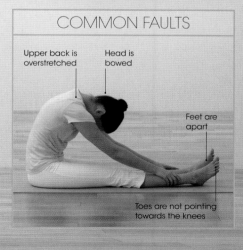

Upper back is overstretched

Head is bowed

Feet are apart

Toes are not pointing towards the knees

Forward Bend
Intermediate and Advanced

Progress in Forward Bend depends on how much you can lengthen the hamstring muscles at the back of your legs, which then allows the pelvis to tilt forwards at the hip joint.

Start with

1 p96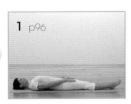

2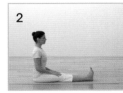

3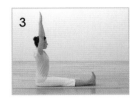

4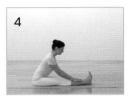

Intermediate

5 Starting from Forward Bend Step 4, if your hands reach your feet, take hold of your big toe in the Classical Foothold (see right).

Keep the back, neck, and head aligned

Bend from the hips and lower back

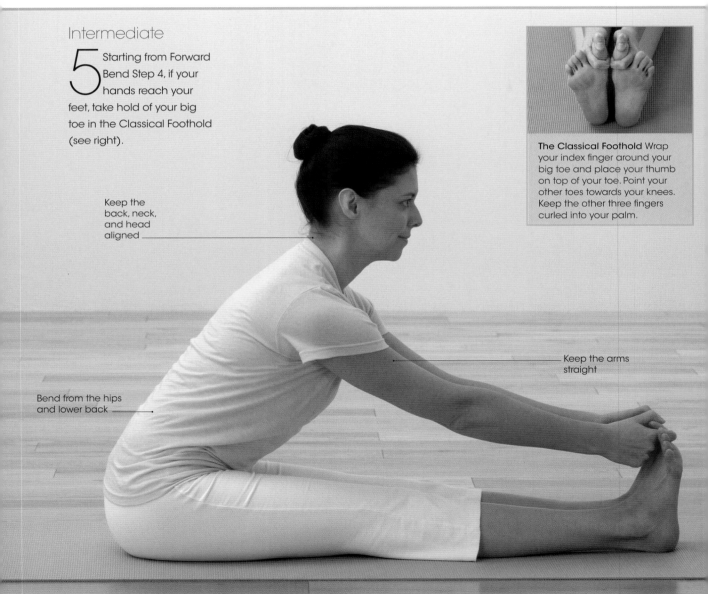

The Classical Foothold Wrap your index finger around your big toe and place your thumb on top of your toe. Point your other toes towards your knees. Keep the other three fingers curled into your palm.

Keep the arms straight

6 On an exhalation, stretch your spine further forwards. Bend your elbows to help you stretch your spine. Repeat 3–4 times, each time holding the pose for a few breaths more. Continue with Step 7 or come back up on an inhalation.

Actively pull the toes towards the head

Keep the back, neck, and head aligned

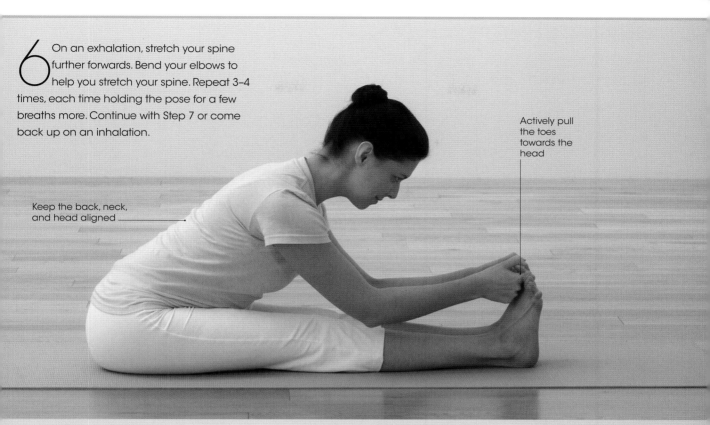

Advanced

7 If you are able to stretch forwards, come into the full pose. On an exhalation, bend farther forwards until your elbows touch the mat and your forehead is resting on your legs. Hold for 1–5 minutes, then come back up on an inhalation. Next, practise Inclined Plane (see p100), then relax with deep abdominal breathing (see p46) for 1–2 minutes in Corpse Pose (see p188).

Rest the chest on the knees

Rest the head between the shins

Rest the abdomen on the thighs

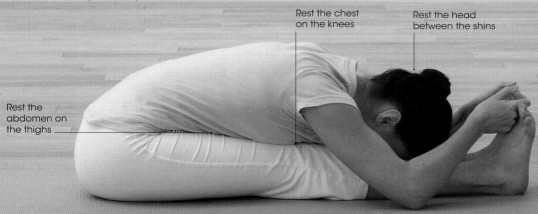

Inclined Plane
All Levels

When you have practised Forward Bend (see pp96–9), practise Inclined Plane as the counterpose. It will help to strengthen the muscles of your arms, legs, and back. Relax afterwards in Corpse Pose (see p188).

1 Sit with your legs stretched straight in front of you and place your hands about 30cm (12in) behind you on the mat. Drop your head backwards, keeping your neck and throat relaxed. Rest on your hands.

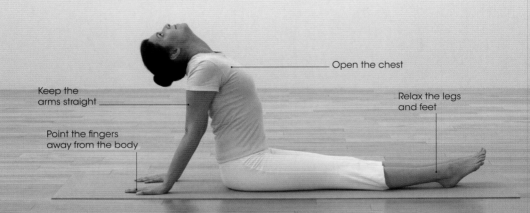

Open the chest

Keep the arms straight

Relax the legs and feet

Point the fingers away from the body

2 Inhale and lift your hips as high as possible. Hold your breath as you gently push your feet into the floor. Exhale and return to Step 1. Repeat twice more. Once you are accustomed to the pose, try to hold it, breathing rhythmically, for up to 30 seconds. Come down by bringing your hips back to the floor.

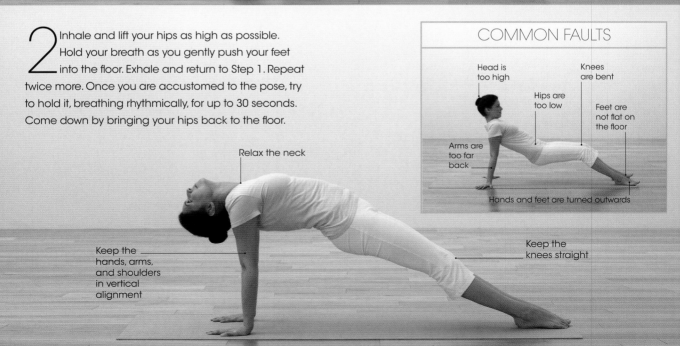

Relax the neck

Keep the hands, arms, and shoulders in vertical alignment

Keep the knees straight

COMMON FAULTS

Head is too high

Knees are bent

Hips are too low

Feet are not flat on the floor

Arms are too far back

Hands and feet are turned outwards

One Leg Up
Intermediate Variation

Starting from Inclined Plane Step 2
(see opposite), inhale and lift your
left leg straight up. Exhale and lower
your leg, then repeat twice more.
Repeat 3 times on the other side.

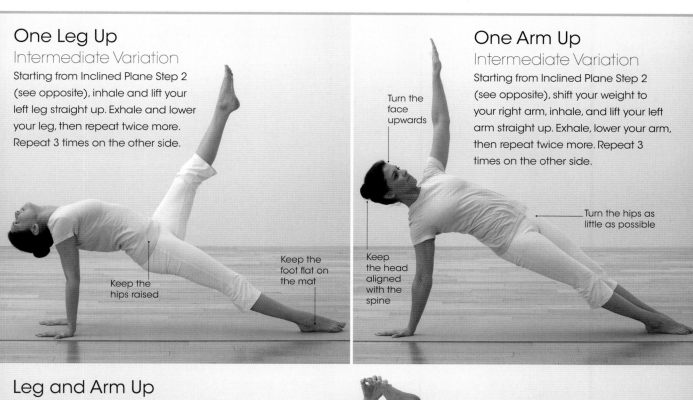

Keep the
hips raised

Keep the
foot flat on
the mat

One Arm Up
Intermediate Variation

Starting from Inclined Plane Step 2
(see opposite), shift your weight to
your right arm, inhale, and lift your left
arm straight up. Exhale, lower your arm,
then repeat twice more. Repeat 3
times on the other side.

Turn the
face
upwards

Turn the hips as
little as possible

Keep
the head
aligned
with the
spine

Leg and Arm Up
Advanced Variation

Starting from Inclined Plane Step 2 (see
opposite), inhale and lift your right leg.
On the next inhalation, lift your left arm.
Keeping firmly balanced on your right arm
and left leg, slowly move your chest
towards the raised leg and catch
hold of your raised foot. After a few
deep breaths, release. Repeat on
the other side.

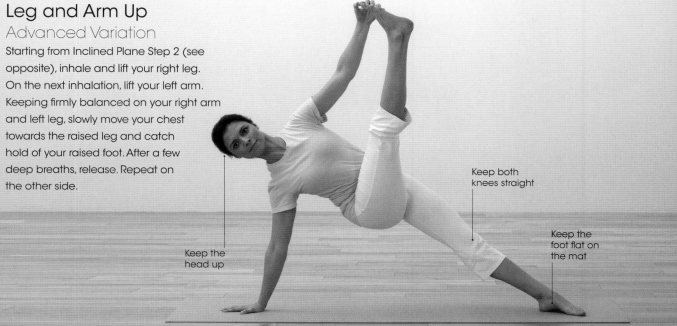

Keep both
knees straight

Keep the
foot flat on
the mat

Keep the
head up

Forward Bend
Variations

When practising Forward Bend variations, practise the counterpose – Inclined Plane (see p100) – between each variation and after you practise your last variation, then relax in Corpse Pose (see p188).

Single Leg Forward Bend
Beginner

1 Sit with your legs stretched out in front of you, then bend your right knee and place the sole of your right foot against your left thigh. Inhale and raise your arms over your head.

Stretch the fingers up

Look straight ahead

Pull the toes towards the head

2 Exhale, bend from the waist over your left leg, and place your hands on your leg, ankle, or foot. With each exhalation, let your spine move forwards. Aim to rest your abdomen on your thigh, your chest on your knee, and your head on your shin. Hold the pose for 1–3 minutes. Release and repeat on the other side.

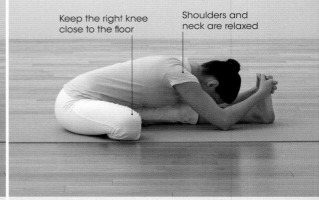

Keep the right knee close to the floor

Shoulders and neck are relaxed

Butterfly
Beginner

1 Sit with your legs stretched out in front of you, then bend your knees, take hold of your feet, and bring them close to your body.

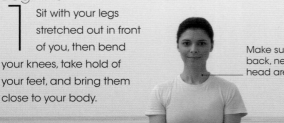

Make sure the back, neck, and head are aligned

Keep the soles of the feet together

2 Rhythmically push your knees down towards the floor, then release so they come back up. Repeat 10–20 times.

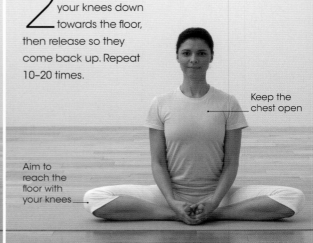

Keep the chest open

Aim to reach the floor with your knees

Half Lotus Forward Bend
Intermediate

1 Sit with your legs stretched out in front of you, then bend your left knee and take your left foot on top of your right thigh, close to your hips. This is Half Lotus. Inhale and raise your arms over your head. If your left knee does not rest on the floor, you should practise only Single Leg Forward Bend (see opposite).

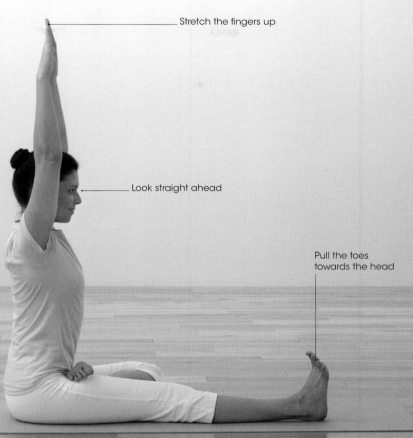

Stretch the fingers up

Look straight ahead

Pull the toes towards the head

2 With an exhalation, bend from the waist over your right leg and reach forwards. Place your hands on your leg or ankle, or hold onto your foot. With each exhalation, allow your spine to move forwards more. Hold the pose for 1–3 minutes. Release and repeat on the other side.

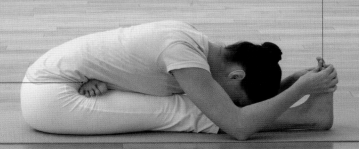

Actively pull the toes towards the head

Breathe deeply, pushing the abdomen against the foot

Forward Bend
Variations (continued)

These Forward Bend variations work on the flexion, abduction, and external rotation of the hip joints. They will make everyday sitting, standing, and walking much easier.

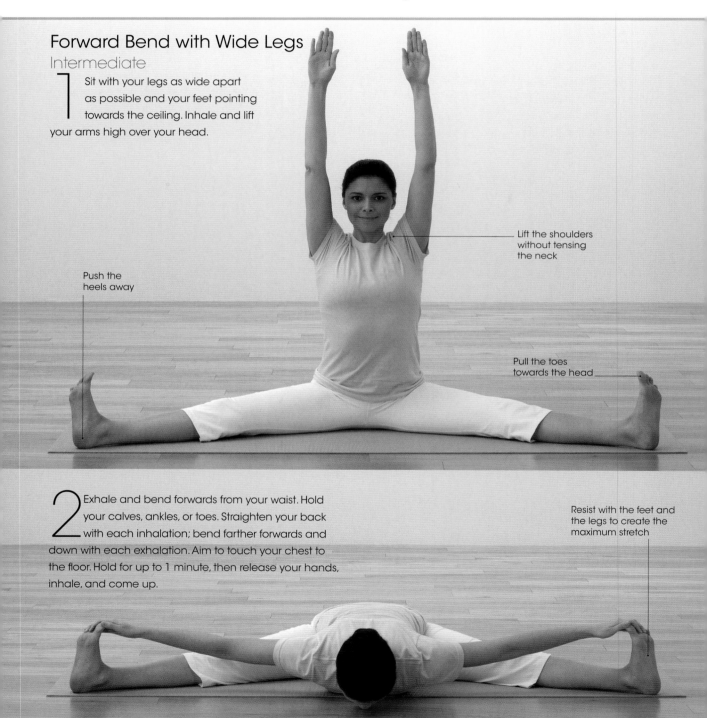

Forward Bend with Wide Legs
Intermediate

1 Sit with your legs as wide apart as possible and your feet pointing towards the ceiling. Inhale and lift your arms high over your head.

Lift the shoulders without tensing the neck

Push the heels away

Pull the toes towards the head

2 Exhale and bend forwards from your waist. Hold your calves, ankles, or toes. Straighten your back with each inhalation; bend farther forwards and down with each exhalation. Aim to touch your chest to the floor. Hold for up to 1 minute, then release your hands, inhale, and come up.

Resist with the feet and the legs to create the maximum stretch

Start with

1 p103

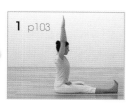

Bound Half Lotus Forward Bend
Advanced

2 Starting from Half Lotus Forward Bend Step 1, bring your left arm behind your back and hold your left foot. Exhale, bend from the waist, and reach forwards to hold the toes of your right foot. Hold the pose for up to 1 minute. Release and repeat on the other side.

Use the Classical Foothold (see p98)

Rest the elbow on the floor

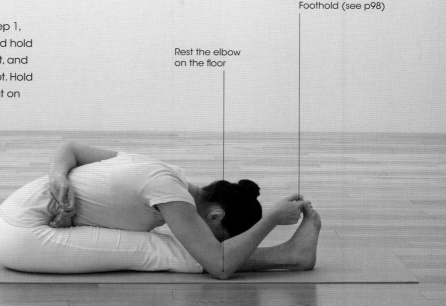

Straight Arm Forward Bend
Advanced

Sitting with your legs outstretched, inhale, raise your arms, then exhale and bend forwards. Put your hands in Prayer Position (see p50) and place your hands, wrists, or forearms on your toes. Hold for up to 1 minute, then release.

Keep upper arms by ears

Keep elbows straight

Bend forwards from the hip joint

Forward Bend
Variations (continued)

These Forward Bend variations are good examples of how asanas prepare you for the meditative sitting poses (see p203). They help you to gain the necessary flexibility, strength, and balance.

Tortoise
Advanced

1 Sit with legs apart, knees bent, and feet flat on the floor, as close to your body as possible. Bend forwards and place your arms under your bent knees, reaching as far back as possible.

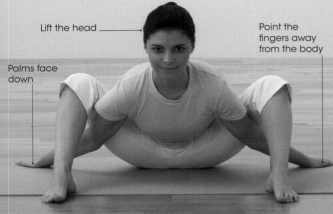

Lift the head

Point the fingers away from the body

Palms face down

2 With an exhalation, bend forwards from the waist until your chin, forehead, or chest touches the floor. Push your heels forwards and straighten your knees as much as possible. Hold, breathing rhythmically, for up to 1 minute, then slide your legs closer to you until you can take your arms out from underneath your knees.

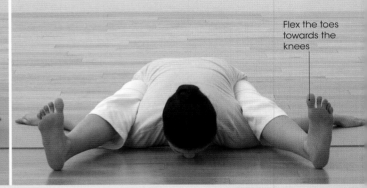

Flex the toes towards the knees

Seated One Leg Raise
Advanced

Sit with your legs stretched out in front of you, then bend your right leg and place your right foot in front of your body. Bend forwards, reach for your left leg, and pull it straight up, holding onto your calf, ankle, or toes. Hold, breathing rhythmically, for up to 1 minute. Release and repeat on the other side.

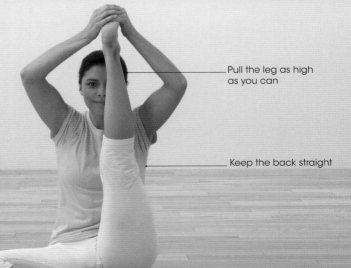

Pull the leg as high as you can

Keep the back straight

Start with

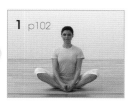

1 p102

Seated Two Leg Raise
Advanced

2 Before beginning, make sure there is enough space behind you in case you lose your balance and roll backwards. Starting from Butterfly Step 1, inhale and pull both legs straight up in front of you. Clasp your calves, ankles, or toes. Hold, breathing rhythmically, for 30 seconds, then release.

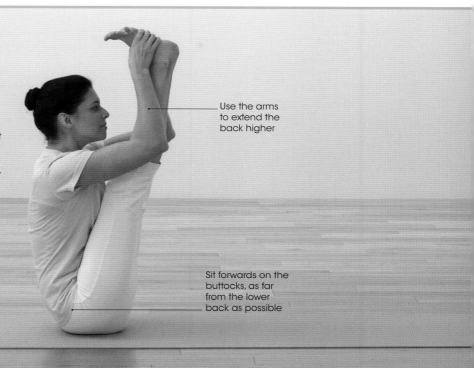

Use the arms to extend the back higher

Sit forwards on the buttocks, as far from the lower back as possible

Lateral Bend with Twist
Advanced

Sit with legs apart, feet pointing upwards. Place your right foot in front of your groin or against your left thigh. Inhale, stretch both arms up, and twist to the right. Exhale and bend sideways. Catch your big left toe in the Classical Foothold (see p98) and place your right hand on the outside of your left foot. Hold, breathing rhythmically, for up to 1 minute. Release and repeat on the other side.

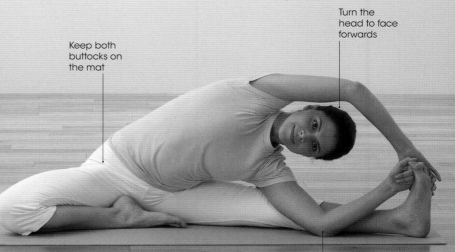

Keep both buttocks on the mat

Turn the head to face forwards

Place the elbow on the knee or on the floor

One Foot to Head
All Levels

Try these challenging poses according to your level of ability. Rest afterwards in Corpse Pose (see p188) so the muscles of your pelvis and lower back can relax completely.

Beginner

1 Starting from a sitting position, bring your left foot close to your body. Lift your right leg and cradle your right knee and foot. With a rhythmical exhalation and inhalation, gently rock to and fro to twist the spine and open the hip joint. Repeat 4 times, then repeat on the other side. Continue with Step 2 or relax.

Keep the back straight

Keep the calf parallel to the floor

Intermediate

2 Return to the sitting position as before, then pull your right foot into the middle of your chest. On an inhalation, straighten your back, and on an exhalation, bring your foot closer to your chest. Hold for up to 1 minute, breathing rhythmically. Repeat on the other side. Continue with Step 3 or relax.

Keep the shoulders even

Keep the foot close to the body

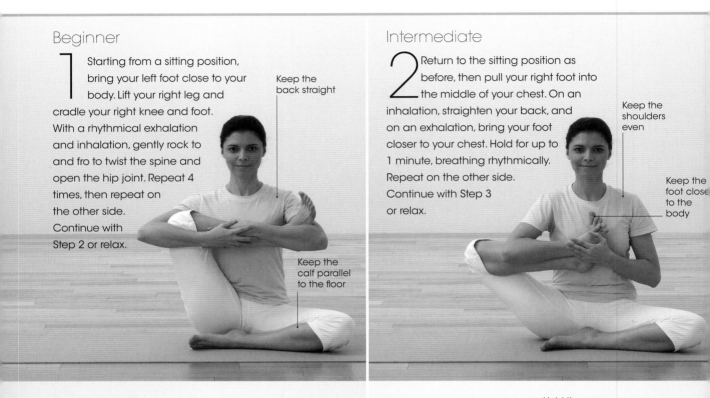

Advanced

3 Return to the sitting position as before. Use both hands to pull your right knee over your right shoulder. Breathing deeply, hold for up to 1 minute. Repeat on the other side.

Take the knee over the shoulder

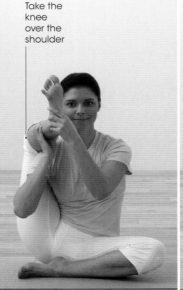

4 Return to the sitting position as before. Raise your left arm and lift up your right foot. Take your right hand to the floor. Breathing rhythmically, hold for up to 30 seconds. Repeat on the other side.

Hold the foot firmly

Raise the arm

Use the hand on the floor for balance

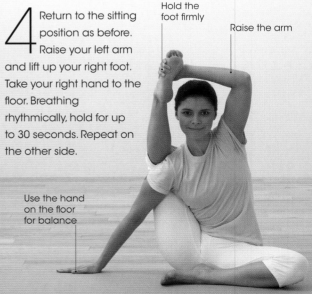

5 To come into the full pose, return to the sitting position as before. Bend your head forwards and use your left hand to pull your right foot behind your head. Take your head back against your right foot and place your hands in Prayer Position (see p50) in front of your chest. Hold for a few rhythmical breaths, then release the pose by following Steps 4 and 3 in that order. Repeat on the other side.

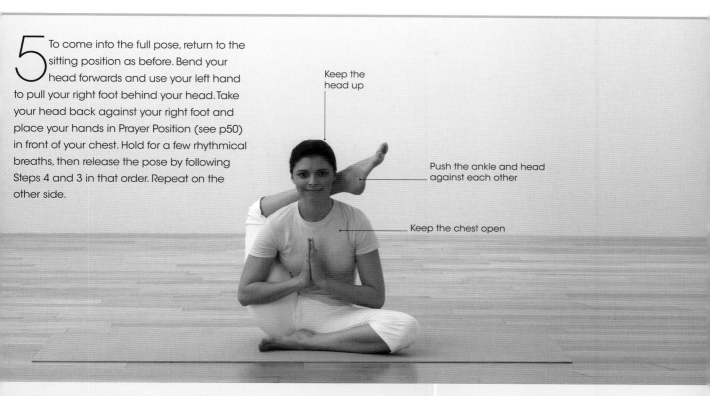

Keep the head up

Push the ankle and head against each other

Keep the chest open

Lying Down Leg Behind Head
Advanced Variation

Starting from One Foot to Head Step 5 (see above), stretch out your left leg and slowly lie down on the mat. Hold for a few rhythmical breaths, then take hold of your right foot with your right hand, and carefully release your right leg. Repeat on the other side.

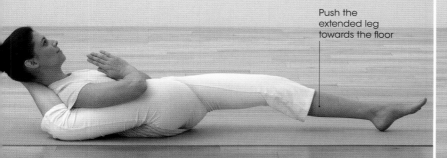

Push the extended leg towards the floor

Both Legs Behind Head
Advanced Variation

Starting from Lying Down Leg Behind Head (see left), take your left foot behind your head. Lock your left foot with the right. Clasp your hands under your lower back. Hold for a few rhythmical breaths, then unlock your feet and roll out of the pose. Repeat on the other side.

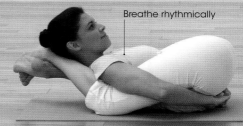

Breathe rhythmically

Shooting Bow
Advanced

These variations will help you improve your Forward Bend (see pp96–9). After practising Shooting Bow, return to Forward Bend step 5, then practise Inclined Plane (see p100), then relax in Corpse pose (see p188).

Start with

1 p96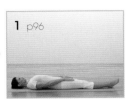

2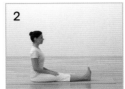

3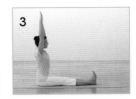

4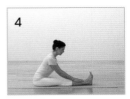

5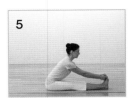

6 Starting from Forward Bend Step 5, inhale and bend your right knee, pulling your right foot back and up as close to your right ear as possible. Keep your raised elbow as high as possible. After a few breaths, release your foot, then repeat on the other side.

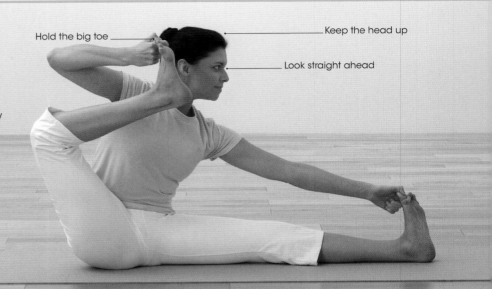

Hold the big toe

Keep the head up

Look straight ahead

Diagonal Shooting Bow
Variation

Starting from Forward Bend Step 5, take your left arm on top of your right so each hand is holding the opposite foot. Inhale and pull your left foot towards your right ear. After a few breaths, release your leg, then repeat, crossing your arms the other way and pulling your right foot towards your left ear.

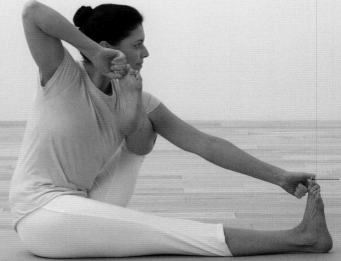

Hold the big toe of the opposite foot

"Asanas give strength. Pranayama gives lightness of body. Meditation gives perception of the Self and leads to freedom or final beatitude." Swami Sivananda

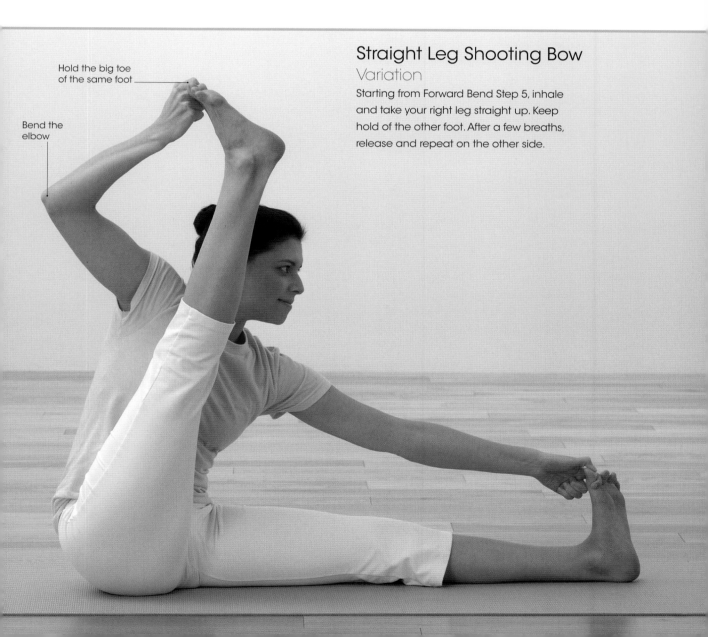

Hold the big toe of the same foot

Bend the elbow

Straight Leg Shooting Bow
Variation

Starting from Forward Bend Step 5, inhale and take your right leg straight up. Keep hold of the other foot. After a few breaths, release and repeat on the other side.

Splits
Advanced

Splits and its variations open up the hip and shoulder joints, as well as the solar plexus area in the abdomen, allowing prana (see p178) to flow. Relax afterwards in Corpse Pose (see p188).

Splits

Kneel down and take your left leg forwards Breathe slowly as you place your hands either side of your body to help you balance, then straighten your right leg behind and push your left heel farther away to deepen the split. If you are flexible enough to sit down, take your hands into Prayer Position (see p50) in front of your chest. Hold for a few breaths then, pressing your hands against the mat, release the pose by bending both legs. Repeat on the other side.

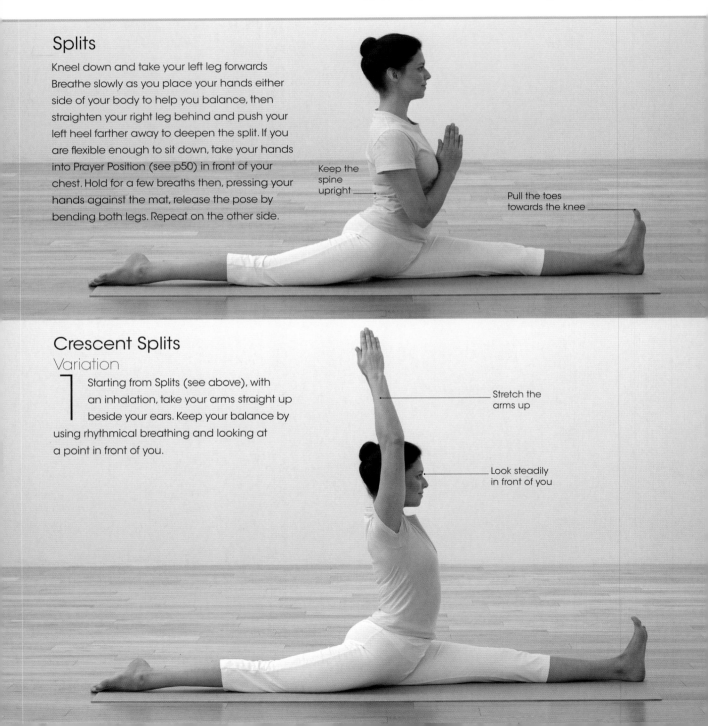

Keep the spine upright

Pull the toes towards the knee

Crescent Splits
Variation

1. Starting from Splits (see above), with an inhalation, take your arms straight up beside your ears. Keep your balance by using rhythmical breathing and looking at a point in front of you.

Stretch the arms up

Look steadily in front of you

2 Still keeping your arms straight, inhale and arch your upper body backwards. Hold for a few breaths, then bring your arms down and release the pose as for Splits (see opposite). Repeat on the other side, release.

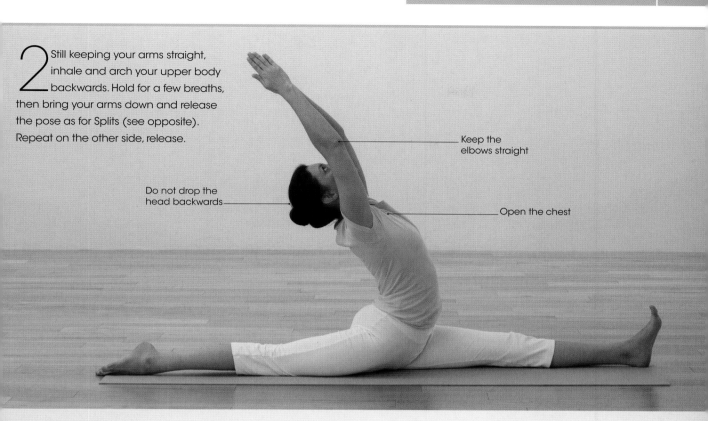

Keep the elbows straight

Do not drop the head backwards

Open the chest

Pigeon Splits
Variation

Starting from Crescent Splits Step 2 (see above), breathe rhythmically as you bend your right knee and catch hold of your right foot with both hands. Hold for a few breaths, then release your hold on your foot and release the pose as for Splits (see opposite). Repeat on the other side.

Try to bring the head to the foot

Avoid twisting the spine

Balance on both legs

Lotus
Advanced

Lotus gives you a stable base so you can keep your back aligned without much effort. The various Lotus positions allow a free flow of prana (see p178). Relax afterwards in Corpse Pose (see p188).

1 Sit cross-legged, then lift your left foot on top of your right thigh, taking the foot as close to your right hip as possible. If necessary, place a small pillow under your sitting bones. Breathe slowly and meditatively.

2 Lift your right foot on top of your left thigh and rest your hands on your knees in Chin Mudra position (see p204). Hold the pose, breathing slowly and meditatively, for 1 minute, then release first the right foot, then the left. Repeat with your legs folded the other way.

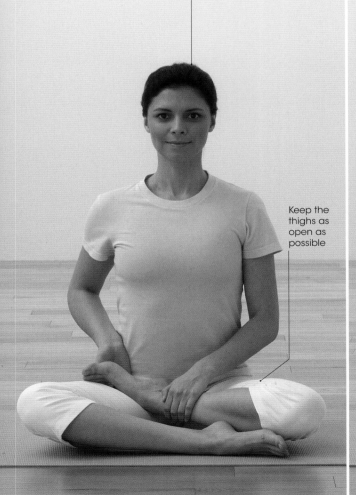

Imagine an invisible thread connecting the top of the head to the ceiling

Keep the thighs as open as possible

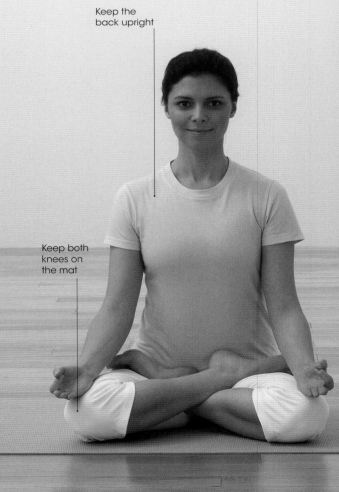

Keep the back upright

Keep both knees on the mat

Lotus Balance
Variation

Starting from Lotus Step 2 (see opposite), lie on your back. Place your arms under your body with your palms under your buttocks. Inhale, contract your abdominal muscles, and raise first your head and chest, then your knees. Hold, breathing deeply, for up to 30 seconds. Bring your knees down and carefully remove your arms and lie back down. Repeat with your legs folded the other way.

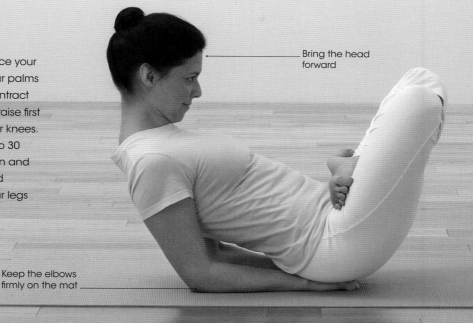

Bring the head forward

Keep the elbows firmly on the mat

Lying Fish
Variation

Starting from Lotus Step 2 (see opposite), lie on your abdomen. Fold your arms and rest your forehead on them. Hold, breathing very slowly and quietly, for up to 1 minute. Come out of the pose by pushing on your elbows and swinging your legs forwards to return to Lotus Step 2. Unfold your legs, then repeat with your legs folded the other way. Release and relax in Child's Pose (see p191).

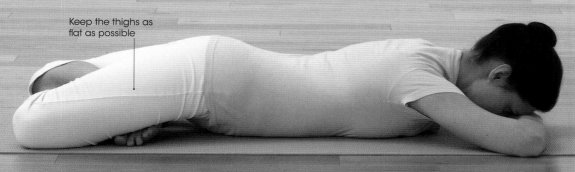

Keep the thighs as flat as possible

6 Cobra
Bujangasana

Like a cobra with its hood raised, in Bhujangasana you arch your head and trunk gracefully upwards. Backward bending against the pull of gravity is the most efficient way to develop a strong back. After Cobra you can either relax on your abdomen (see p190) or stretch back into the counterpose, Child's Pose (see p191).

BENEFITS

PHYSICAL
• Tones the deep and superficial muscles of the back.
• Increases the blood supply to the ligaments of the spine and the vertebrae.
• Removes any tension from overworked back muscles.

• Relieves kyphosis – exaggerated thoracic curvature (see p29).
• Massages the abdominal organs.
• Combats constipation.
• Tones the ovaries and uterus and alleviates menstrual problems.

MENTAL
• By requiring you to focus fully on contracting the muscles in your neck and upper back, Cobra helps to develop your powers of concentration.

Cobra
Beginner and Intermediate

Beginner

1 Lie on your abdomen, keeping your legs straight and your toes together. Point your toes, take your forehead to the mat, and bring your hands alongside your chest, palms face down.

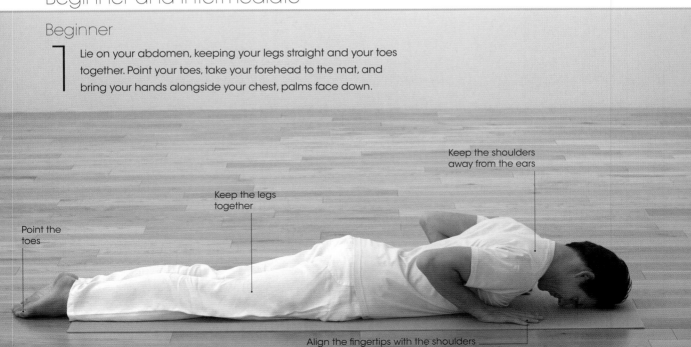

Keep the shoulders away from the ears

Keep the legs together

Point the toes

Align the fingertips with the shoulders

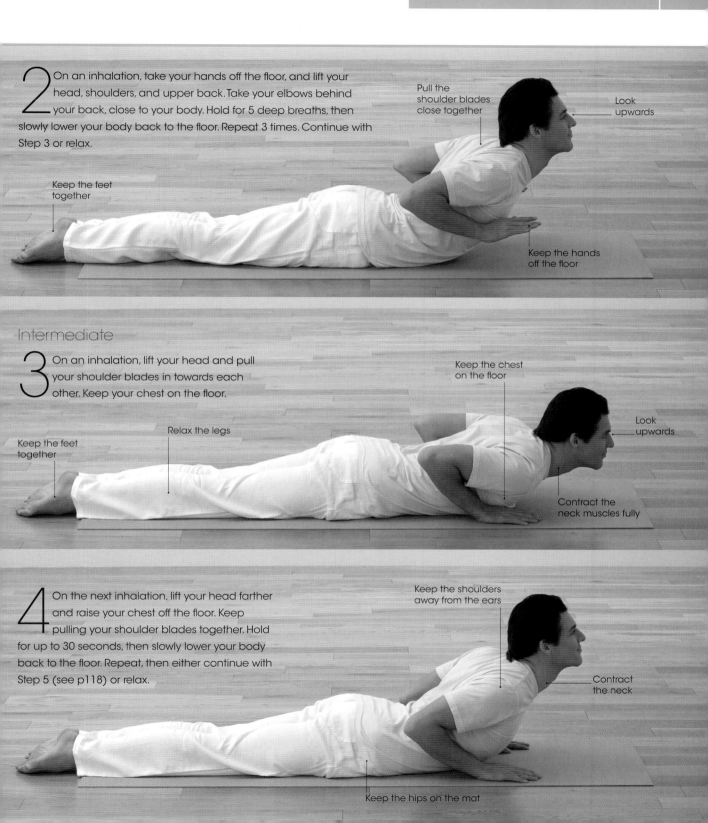

2 On an inhalation, take your hands off the floor, and lift your head, shoulders, and upper back. Take your elbows behind your back, close to your body. Hold for 5 deep breaths, then slowly lower your body back to the floor. Repeat 3 times. Continue with Step 3 or relax.

Pull the shoulder blades close together

Look upwards

Keep the feet together

Keep the hands off the floor

Intermediate

3 On an inhalation, lift your head and pull your shoulder blades in towards each other. Keep your chest on the floor.

Keep the chest on the floor

Relax the legs

Look upwards

Keep the feet together

Contract the neck muscles fully

4 On the next inhalation, lift your head farther and raise your chest off the floor. Keep pulling your shoulder blades together. Hold for up to 30 seconds, then slowly lower your body back to the floor. Repeat, then either continue with Step 5 (see p118) or relax.

Keep the shoulders away from the ears

Contract the neck

Keep the hips on the mat

Cobra
Advanced

Working at a desk encourages rounded shoulders and a collapsed chest, which impairs breathing and depresses your mood. Daily practice of Cobra, at any level, can help to rectify these problems.

Start with

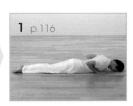
1 p.116

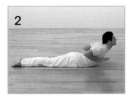
2

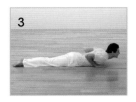
3

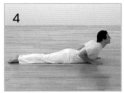
4

5 To come into the full pose, start from Cobra Step 4. On an inhalation, arch your head, neck, and upper back as much as possible. Keep your legs together and make sure that your shoulder blades are pulled backwards and away from your ears. Hold for up to 1 minute, then lower your body back to the floor. Take a few deep breaths, then repeat.

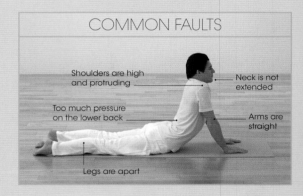

COMMON FAULTS

Shoulders are high and protruding

Neck is not extended

Too much pressure on the lower back

Arms are straight

Legs are apart

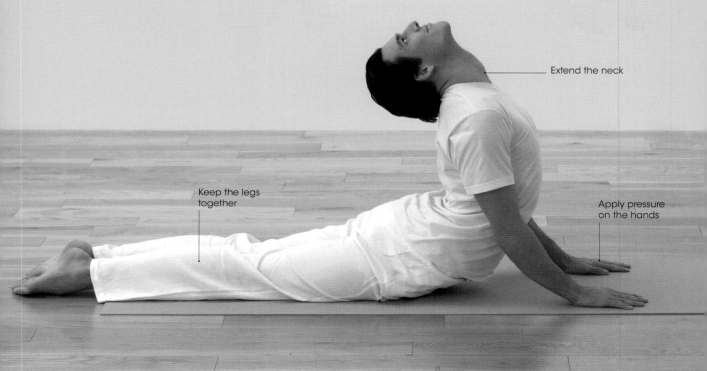

Extend the neck

Keep the legs together

Apply pressure on the hands

Start with

1 p116

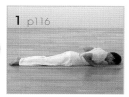

Hands Clasped
Intermediate Variation

2 Starting from Cobra Step 1, take your arms behind your back, straighten them, and clasp your hands together.

Relax the legs

Clasp the hands

Relax the neck and shoulders

3 With an inhalation, lift your head, arms, and chest off the floor. Hold for up to 30 seconds, then lower your body back to the floor. Take a few deep breaths, then repeat.

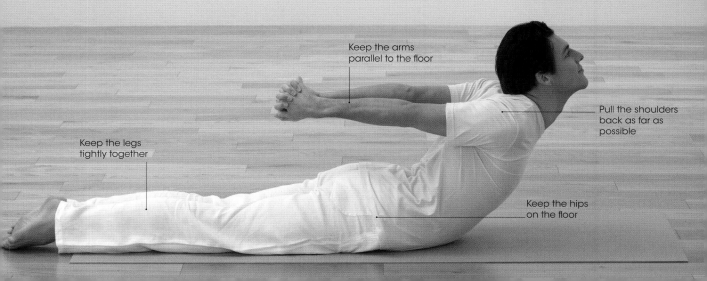

Keep the arms parallel to the floor

Pull the shoulders back as far as possible

Keep the legs tightly together

Keep the hips on the floor

Cobra
Variations (continued)

King Cobra majestically combines contraction of your neck and of the muscles of your upper back with a complete backward bend of your spine. An added benefit is an increase in your lung capacity.

Start with
1 p116
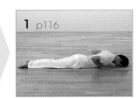

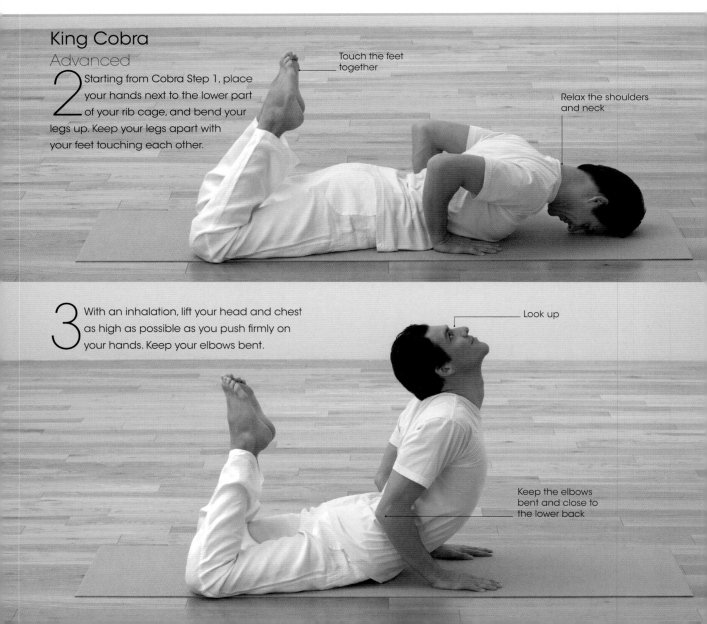

King Cobra
Advanced

2 Starting from Cobra Step 1, place your hands next to the lower part of your rib cage, and bend your legs up. Keep your legs apart with your feet touching each other.

Touch the feet together

Relax the shoulders and neck

3 With an inhalation, lift your head and chest as high as possible as you push firmly on your hands. Keep your elbows bent.

Look up

Keep the elbows bent and close to the lower back

4 With another inhaltion, lift your head and chest even higher. Straighten your arms completely and bring your feet to your head. Hold for up to 30 seconds, then take your feet from your head, and lower your body back to the floor. Take a few deep breaths, then repeat.

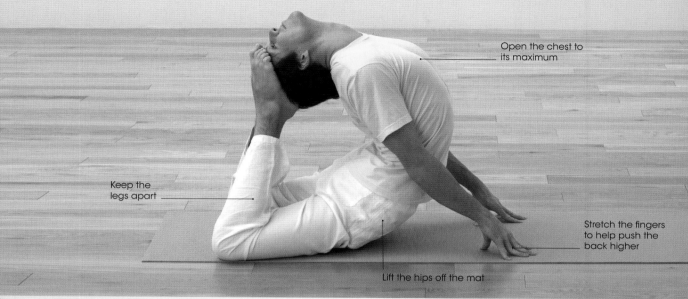

Open the chest to its maximum

Keep the legs apart

Stretch the fingers to help push the back higher

Lift the hips off the mat

King Cobra Knee Hold
Advanced

Starting from King Cobra Step 4 (see above), lift one hand and catch your knee. Find your balance, then catch your other knee with the other hand. Hold for a few breaths, replace your hands in front of you, as in King Cobra Step 4, then lower your body back to the floor. Take a few deep breaths, then repeat.

Pull the shoulders back as far as possible

Hold the knees firmly

Balance on the thighs

7 Locust
Salabhasana

Unlike the other asanas, which are done slowly, you achieve Locust by making a single powerful muscle contraction, similar to that of a locust jumping. This simultaneously brings together thought, breath, movement, and prana – vital energy (see p178). After Locust, stretch back into Child's Pose (see p191) or relax on your front (see p190).

BENEFITS

PHYSICAL
• Strengthens the muscles of the arms, shoulders, abdomen, lower back, thighs, and legs.
• Tones the liver, pancreas, and kidneys.
• Improves the appetite.
• Relieves constipation.

MENTAL
• Of all the asanas, this pose is the one that works most on developing will power. According to Swami Vishnudevananda, exercising will power makes one's thoughts pure and powerful and is the main goal of the practice of asanas. Strong will power also lifts your energy levels from inertia (tamas, see p212) to harmony (satva, see p212).

Locust
All Levels

Beginner

1 Lie on your abdomen with your legs outstretched, heels together, arms under your body, and chin forward on the mat. Place your hands in one of the hand positions (see right), depending on which you find most comfortable. Hand position A is the classical position for this pose.

Hand position A
Interlock the fingers and keep the thumbs together.

Hand position B
Clench the fists and keep the thumbs together.

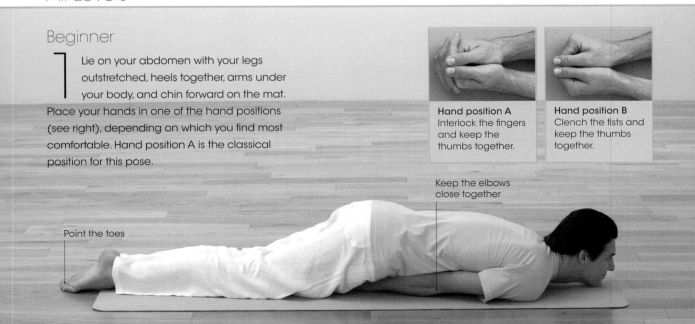

Keep the elbows close together

Point the toes

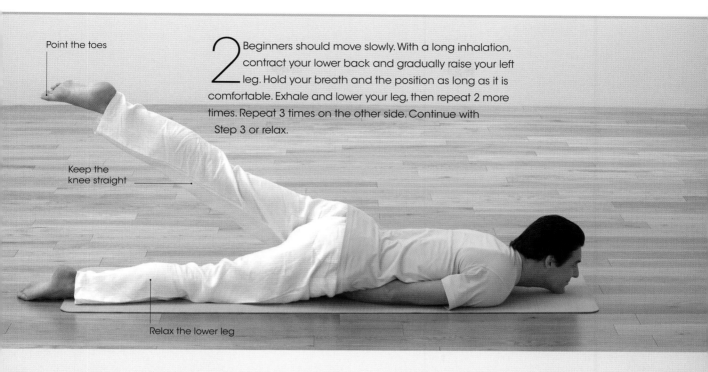

Point the toes

2 Beginners should move slowly. With a long inhalation, contract your lower back and gradually raise your left leg. Hold your breath and the position as long as it is comfortable. Exhale and lower your leg, then repeat 2 more times. Repeat 3 times on the other side. Continue with Step 3 or relax.

Keep the knee straight

Relax the lower leg

Intermediate and Advanced

3 To come into the full pose, on a quick, strong inhalation, contract your lower back, push on your arms, and swing both legs up as high as possible. Hold your breath as long as is comfortable, then exhale and lower your legs. Repeat 2 more times.

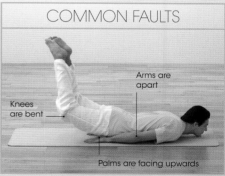

COMMON FAULTS

Arms are apart

Knees are bent

Palms are facing upwards

Point the toes

Keep the legs straight

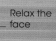

Relax the face

Locust
Variations

The Boat variations are very efficient. You contract your back muscles strongly without putting much pressure on your vertebrae. For maximum benefit, go into and come out of these poses very slowly.

Boat
Beginner

1 Lie face down on the mat with your arms stretched out in front of you and your feet extended behind. Rest your forehead on the floor and breathe deeply in your abdomen. Exhale completely.

2 On an inhalation, simultaneously lift both your arms and legs as high as possible. You may hold your breath or take a few deep breaths in your abdomen. Exhale and release. Repeat up to 3 times.

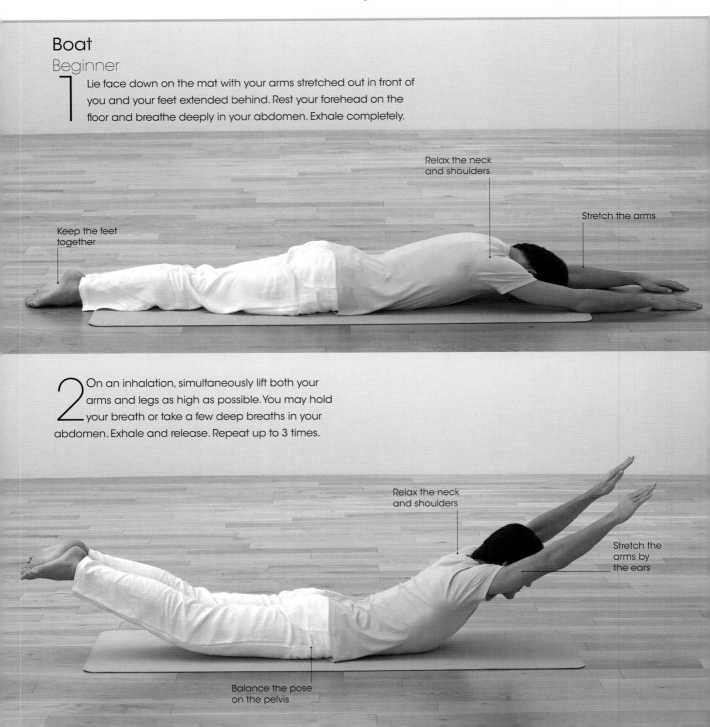

Relax the neck and shoulders

Stretch the arms

Keep the feet together

Relax the neck and shoulders

Stretch the arms by the ears

Balance the pose on the pelvis

Boat with Interlock
Beginner

1 Lie face down on the mat with your feet extended behind you and your forehead on the floor. Take your arms behind your back and hold onto your elbows. Exhale completely.

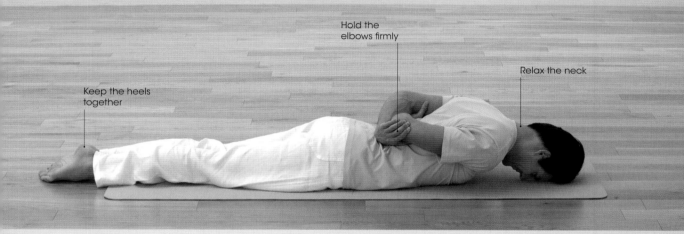

Hold the elbows firmly

Relax the neck

Keep the heels together

2 On an inhalation, lift your legs, head, and chest as high as possible. You may hold your breath or take a few deep breaths. Exhale and release. Repeat up to 3 times.

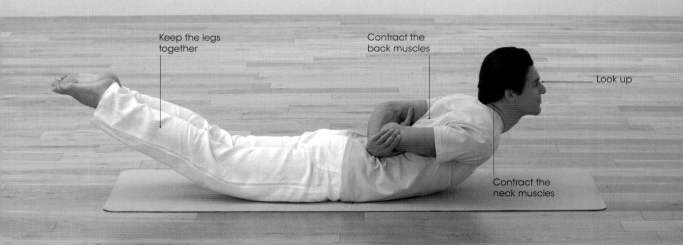

Keep the legs together

Contract the back muscles

Look up

Contract the neck muscles

Locust
Variations (continued)

These Locust variations require regular practice. This will enable you to contract your lower back muscles fast and strongly enough to bring your legs up higher than in Intermediate Locust.

Start with

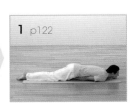

1 p122

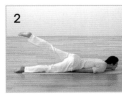

2

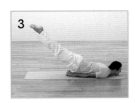

3

High Legs
Advanced

3 Starting from Locust Step 3, inhale and swing your legs up as quickly as you can, adding a strong push with your arms against the floor. Hold for a few breaths, then come out of the pose by slowly releasing the contraction of your back and resisting with your arms. Take a few deep breaths, then repeat. Continue with Feet to Head (see right) or relax.

Keep the legs straight

Push the hands and arms firmly into the mat

Feet to Head
Advanced

Starting from High Legs (see left), focus on taking long exhalations as you bend your knees and lower your feet as close to your head as possible. Hold for a few breaths, then come out of the pose by slowly releasing the contraction of your back and resisting with your arms. Take a few deep breaths, then repeat.

Keep the legs apart

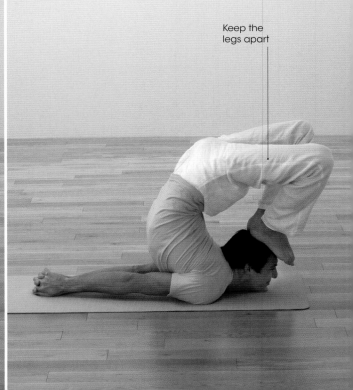

Locust in Lotus
Advanced

1 Start by sitting in Lotus (see p114). Take a few complete yogic breaths (see p181).

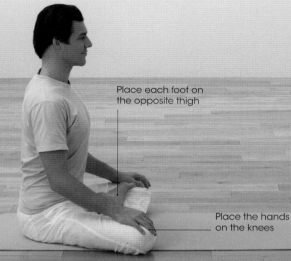

Place each foot on the opposite thigh

Place the hands on the knees

2 Leaning forwards, take your hands onto the floor in front of you and come up onto your knees. Walk your hands forwards until your hands are beneath your shoulders. Breathe slowly and rhythmically.

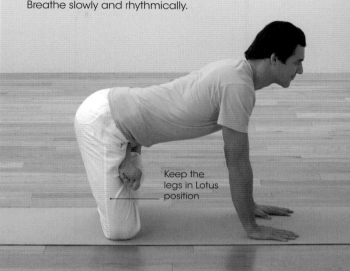

Keep the legs in Lotus position

3 Without releasing your legs, gently lower yourself into a lying position with your arms under your body. Place your hands in one of the hand positions shown on p122, whichever is the most comfortable. Exhale completely.

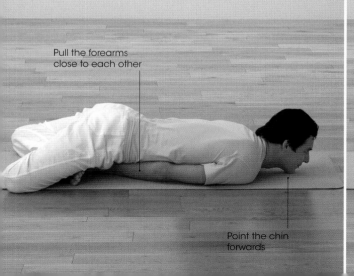

Pull the forearms close to each other

Point the chin forwards

4 Inhale and swing your legs up as quickly and as high as possible. Use the strength of your arms and of your lower back to come up. Hold the pose for a few breaths, then come out by slowly releasing the contraction of your back and resisting with your arms. Repeat, crossing your legs the other way.

Strongly push the hands and arms against the mat

Camel
Beginner and Intermediate

Camel stretches your chest and throat muscles while also strengthening your hamstrings and the muscles of your buttocks. Relax in Child's Pose (see p191) for at least 8 breaths afterwards.

Beginner

1 Kneel on the mat with your knees and feet hip-width apart, arms by your sides. Breathe slowly and rhythmically.

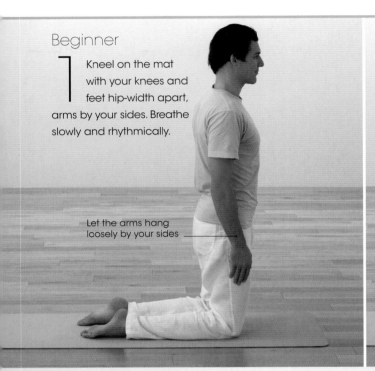

Let the arms hang loosely by your sides

2 Support your lower back with both hands. Inhale and slowly bend backwards, taking your head back first, then your shoulders and chest, and finally your lower back. Hold for up to 30 seconds, breathing slowly and rhythmically. Continue with Step 3 or come out of the pose by inhaling, contracting your abdomen, and lifting your torso back up.

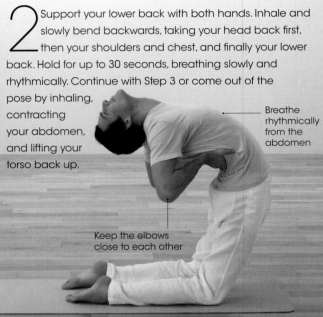

Breathe rhythmically from the abdomen

Keep the elbows close to each other

Intermediate

3 To come into the full pose, breathe slowly as you take your hands, one at a time, from your back to your ankles. Push your pelvis forwards by contracting your buttocks and the backs of your thighs. Hold for up to 30 seconds, breathing slowly and rhythmically from your abdomen. On an inhalation, contract your abdomen and lift your torso back up, then repeat.

Lift the chest

Keep the pelvis forwards

There should be only a minimum of weight on the hands

Diamond
Intermediate and Advanced

Diamond is a complete backward bend, which gives a wonderful stretch to the front of the body and revitalizes the area of the solar plexus. Relax in Child's Pose (see p191) afterwards.

Intermediate

1 Kneel, then sit between your heels, taking your arms behind you. Slowly lower your body onto your elbows, then come into a lying position with your arms behind your head, each hand clasping the opposite elbow. Hold for up to 30 seconds, breathing slowly and rhythmically in your abdomen. Continue with Step 2 or come out of the pose by placing your elbows next to your lower back and pushing yourself up. Then extend your legs in front of you.

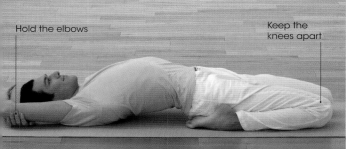

Hold the elbows

Keep the knees apart

Advanced

2 Place your palms flat on the mat as close to your shoulders as possible. Inhale, push on your arms, and place the top of your head on the floor.

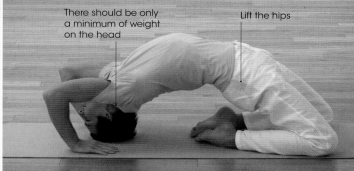

There should be only a minimum of weight on the head

Lift the hips

3 To come into the full pose, with a deep inhalation and another push of your arms, take your head closer to your feet. Move your hands to your feet and push your elbows firmly into the ground. Hold for up to 30 seconds, then release by walking your hands away from your body and lowering your neck to the mat. Repeat, then push yourself up by placing your elbows next to your lower back. Extend your legs in front of you.

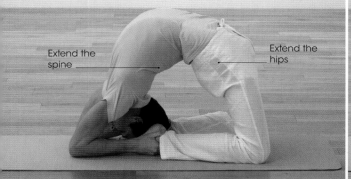

Extend the spine

Extend the hips

Hands on Thighs
Advanced Variation

Starting from Diamond Step 2, with an inhalation, slowly lift one arm at a time and place your hands on your thighs so you are balancing on your head and legs. Hold for a few breaths, then release by returning to Diamond Step 2, then lower your neck to the mat. Repeat, then push yourself up by placing your elbows next to your lower back. Extend your legs in front of you.

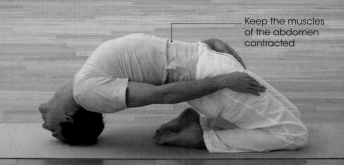

Keep the muscles of the abdomen contracted

Pigeon
All Levels

Holding onto your foot by extending your arms over your head in a sitting position is a thrilling experience. It stretches your spine completely. Relax afterwards in Child's Pose (see p191).

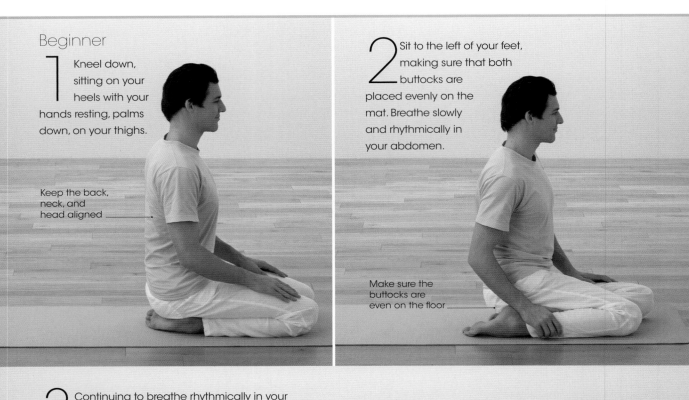

Beginner

1 Kneel down, sitting on your heels with your hands resting, palms down, on your thighs.

Keep the back, neck, and head aligned

2 Sit to the left of your feet, making sure that both buttocks are placed evenly on the mat. Breathe slowly and rhythmically in your abdomen.

Make sure the buttocks are even on the floor

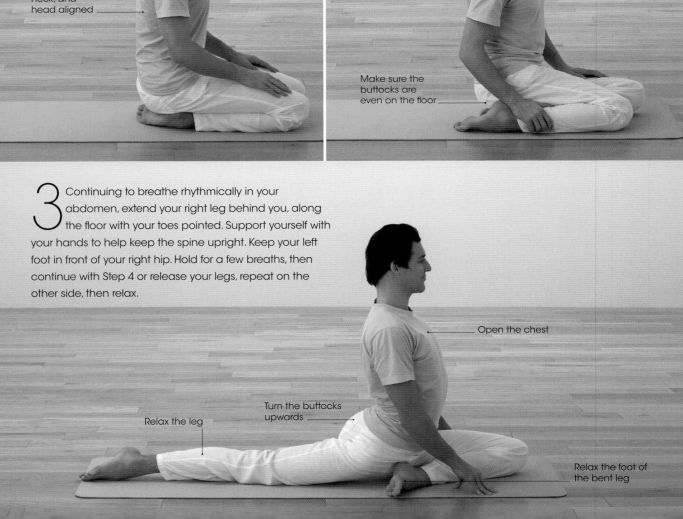

3 Continuing to breathe rhythmically in your abdomen, extend your right leg behind you, along the floor with your toes pointed. Support yourself with your hands to help keep the spine upright. Keep your left foot in front of your right hip. Hold for a few breaths, then continue with Step 4 or release your legs, repeat on the other side, then relax.

Open the chest

Turn the buttocks upwards

Relax the leg

Relax the foot of the bent leg

Intermediate

4 Bend your right knee, reach back with your right hand, and push your right heel against your right buttock. Hold for a few breaths, then continue with Step 5 or repeat on the other side, then relax.

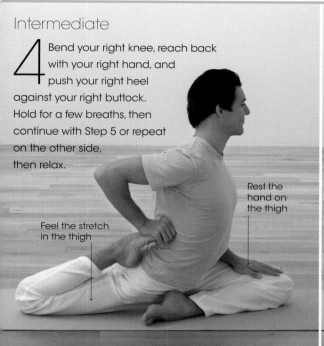

Feel the stretch in the thigh

Rest the hand on the thigh

Advanced

5 Catch the inner edge of your right foot with your right hand. Place your left hand on the floor next to your left hip to help you balance. Keep your breath flowing rhythmically.

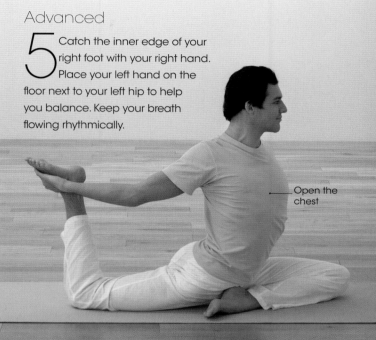

Open the chest

6 Taking your head back, pull your right foot close to your shoulder with your right hand. Continuing to breathe rhythmically, turn your right elbow upwards. Stabilize yourself with your left hand on the mat.

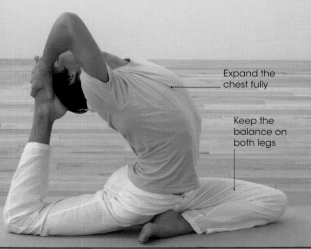

Expand the chest fully

Keep the balance on both legs

7 To come into the full pose, breathe rhythmically to help you balance, bring your left arm over your head, and place your left hand next to your right hand on your right foot. Try to bring your right foot to the top of your head. Hold for a few breaths, then release. Repeat on the other side.

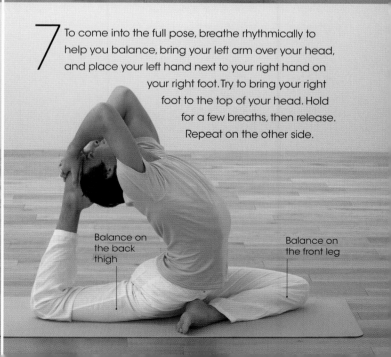

Balance on the back thigh

Balance on the front leg

Crescent Moon
All Levels

This asana stretches the hip flexors (iliopsoas) in the pelvis, which are often shortened due to our sedentary lifestyle, and cause stiffness in the lower back. Relax afterwards in Child's Pose (see p191).

Beginner

1 Kneel on the floor, then take your right foot forwards between your hands. Stretch your left leg back, placing your left knee on the mat. Keep your front calf vertical. Breathe slowly and rhythmically.

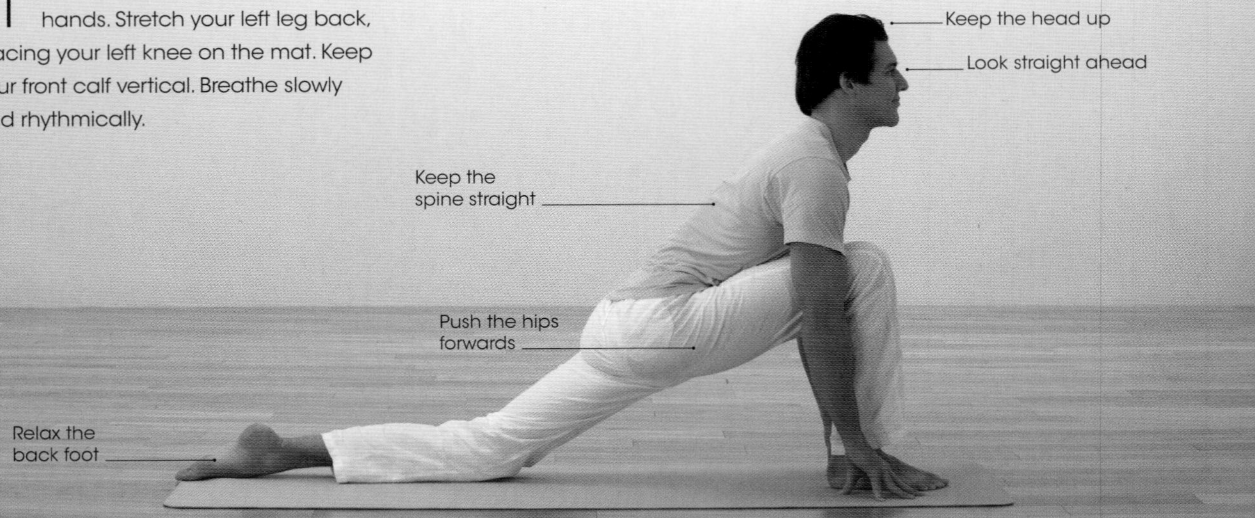

Keep the head up

Look straight ahead

Keep the spine straight

Push the hips forwards

Relax the back foot

2 Inhale and take your hands in front of your chest in Prayer Position (see p50). Keep your back vertical and use your bent leg and the toes of your front foot to help you balance. Hold for a few breaths, then continue with Step 3 or release the pose, repeat on the other side, then relax.

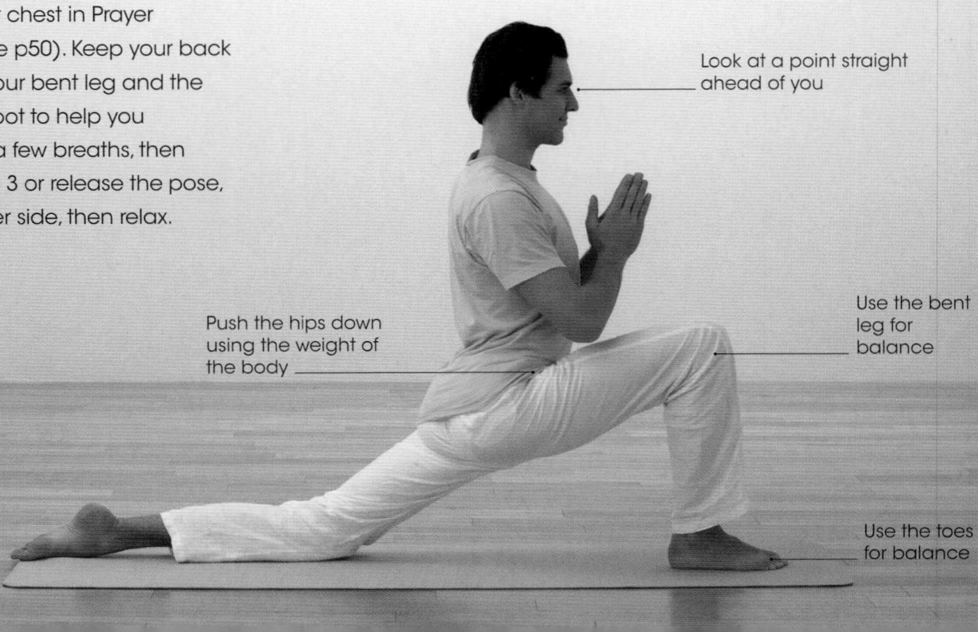

Look at a point straight ahead of you

Push the hips down using the weight of the body

Use the bent leg for balance

Use the toes for balance

Intermediate

3 On an inhalation, take both arms straight up beside your ears. Hold for up to 30 seconds, breathing slowly and rhythmically. On each inhalation, stretch your arms higher; on each exhalation, try to lower your hips to the floor a little more. Continue with Step 4 or release the pose, repeat on the other side, then relax.

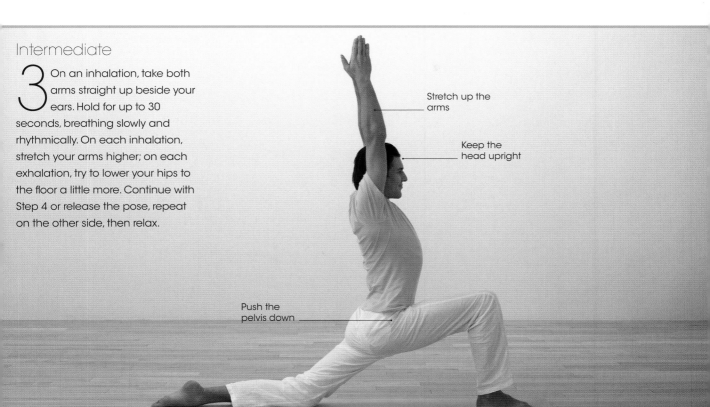

Stretch up the arms

Keep the head upright

Push the pelvis down

Advanced

4 To come into the full pose, on another inhalation, bend backwards from your chest. Hold for up to 30 seconds, then repeat on the other side.

Keep the arms aligned with the ears

Push the pelvis forwards

Feel the stretch in the back thigh

Relax the back foot

8 Bow
Dhanurasana

Bow combines the benefits of Cobra (see pp116–18) and of Locust (see pp122–3). In this pose, the muscles of the legs and back are activated to form the shape of a bow, while the arms are stretched passively like the string of a bow. Relax afterwards in the counterpose, Child's Pose (see p191) for 8 breaths.

BENEFITS

PHYSICAL
- Tones the muscles of the back.
- Maintains the elasticity of the whole spine.
- Counteracts kyphosis – excessive curvature of the upper back (see p29).
- Strengthens the quadriceps muscles in the front of the thighs.
- Alleviates gastrointestinal disorders.
- Energizes digestion.
- Relieves constipation.
- Energizes the female reproductive system.

MENTAL
- Counteracts mental sluggishness and laziness.

Bow
Beginner

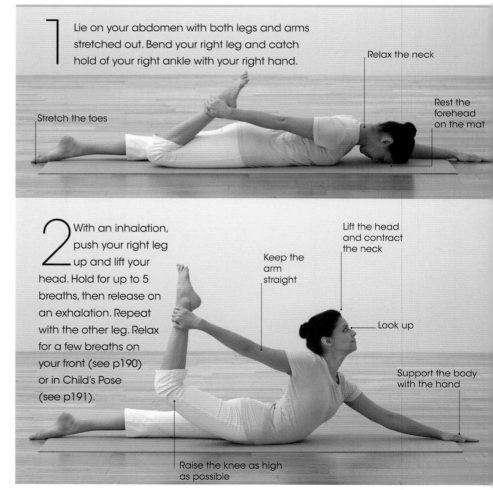

1 Lie on your abdomen with both legs and arms stretched out. Bend your right leg and catch hold of your right ankle with your right hand.

Relax the neck

Rest the forehead on the mat

Stretch the toes

2 With an inhalation, push your right leg up and lift your head. Hold for up to 5 breaths, then release on an exhalation. Repeat with the other leg. Relax for a few breaths on your front (see p190) or in Child's Pose (see p191).

Lift the head and contract the neck

Keep the arm straight

Look up

Support the body with the hand

Raise the knee as high as possible

Bow
Intermediate and Advanced

1 Lie on your abdomen with your knees apart. Bend your legs and catch hold of your ankles.

Relax the toes

Keep the arms straight

Rest the forehead on the mat

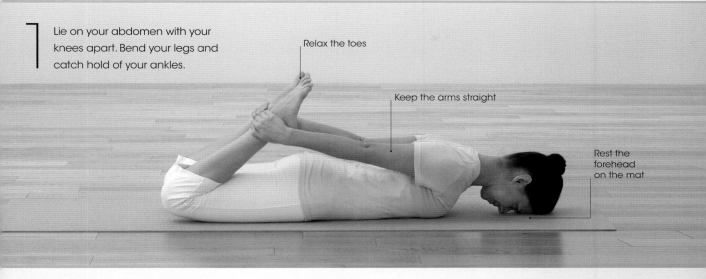

2 To come into the full pose, on an inhalation, push your feet up until your knees come as high off the mat as possible. Lift your head and contract your neck. Hold for 3–6 breaths, then exhale, release your feet, and lower your knees and forehead back to the mat.

Keep the arms straight

COMMON FAULTS

Feet are not actively pushing up

Arms are bent and contracted

Head is not lifted

Only upper part of body is lifted

Feet are held instead of ankles

Keep the shoulders away from the ears

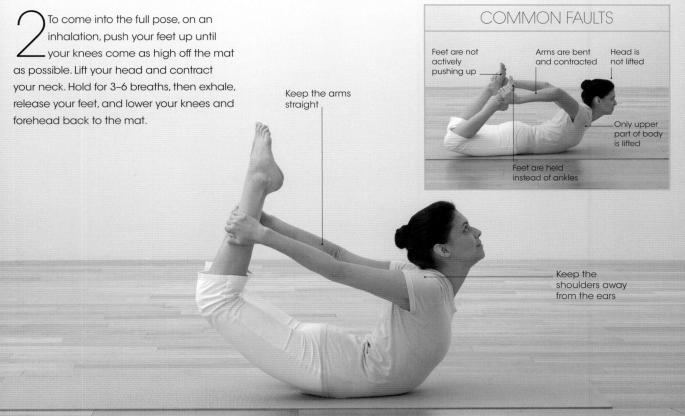

Bow
Variations

These variations bring complete flexibility to the shoulder joints, but require flexible hip and chest muscles. After you have practised them, stretch back into Child's Pose (see p191) to relax.

Start with

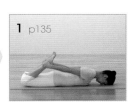

1 p135

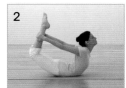

2

Rocking Bow
Intermediate

3 Starting from Bow Step 2, with a strong inhalation, strongly contract your neck and your upper back muscles. Lift your head and chest as high as you can. This creates a backwards rocking motion, shifting your weight from your abdomen to your thighs.

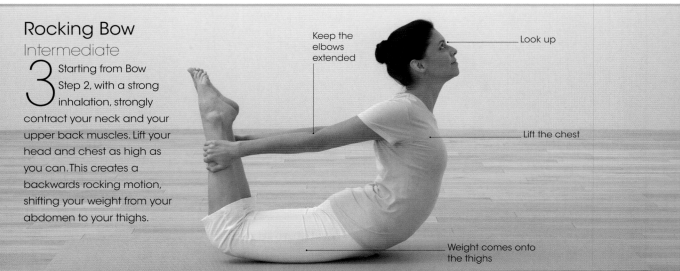

Keep the elbows extended

Look up

Lift the chest

Weight comes onto the thighs

4 With a strong exhalation, use your arms and shoulders to pull your body forwards, moving your weight onto your abdomen and chest. Rock forwards and back 3–6 times, then exhale, release your feet, and lower your knees and forehead back to the mat.

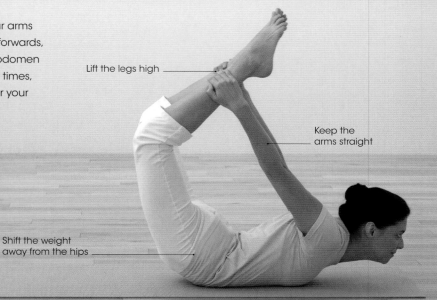

Lift the legs high

Keep the arms straight

Shift the weight away from the hips

One-handed Bow
Advanced

1 Lie on your abdomen, supporting yourself with your bent left arm. Bend your right leg and catch your right foot just below your big toe with your right hand. Keep your left foot stretched behind you.

Support the body with the outstretched arm

Stretch the thigh

2 On an inhalation, pull your right foot closer to your shoulder. Straighten your other arm to help push your chest higher into the backward bend.

Lift the head

Look straight ahead

Keep your balance with the outstretched arm

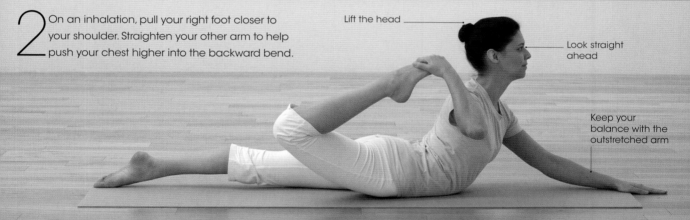

3 Once your foot is close enough to your shoulder, breathe slowly and lift your right elbow, pulling your foot higher up. Hold for a few breaths, then exhale, release your foot, and lower your knee and forehead back to the mat. Repeat on the other side.

Look up

Bend the head backwards

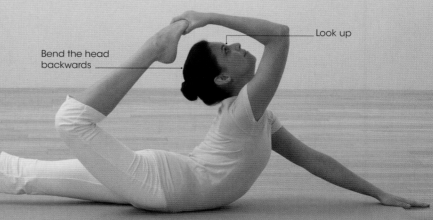

Bow
Variations (continued)

Complete Bow is a truly dynamic pose, to be attempted when you can do One-handed Bow (see p137). It gives you a powerful anterior stretch, all the way from your throat to your knees.

Complete Bow
Advanced

1 Lying on your abdomen, bend both legs and catch hold of each foot, placing your fingers around your big toes and the tops of your feet. Breathe deeply and slowly.

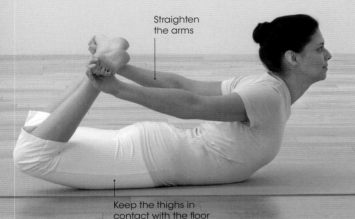

Straighten the arms

Keep the thighs in contact with the floor

2 Rotate your shoulders as you bend your elbows and pull your feet as close to your shoulders as possible. Your thighs will come off the ground. Focus on rhythmical breathing.

Lift the head

Look straight ahead

Keep the knees apart

Thighs lift off the floor

3 Continue breathing slowly. Once your feet are close enough to your shoulders, lift your elbows forwards, in front of your face, pulling your feet even higher. Hold for a few breaths, then exhale, release your feet, and lower your knees and forehead back to the mat.

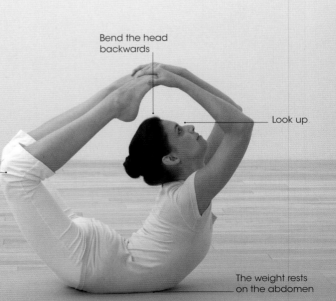

Bend the head backwards

Look up

Extend the knees to help lift the feet

The weight rests on the abdomen

Feet to Head
Advanced

Starting from Complete Bow Step 3 (see opposite), breathe slowly and rhythmically as you continue gently pulling your feet until they touch your forehead. Hold for a few breaths, then exhale, release your feet, and lower your knees and forehead back to the mat.

Keep the knees apart

Extend the neck to the maximum

Contract the arms

Feet to Shoulders
Advanced

Starting from Feet to Head (see above), with slow breathing, try to pull your feet gently on top of your shoulders. This requires great flexibility of the spine and shoulders. Hold for a few breaths, then exhale, release your feet, and lower your knees and forehead back to the mat.

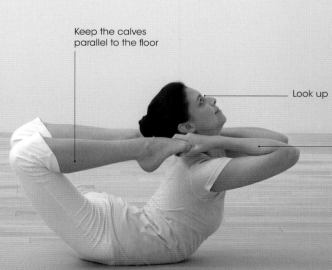

Keep the calves parallel to the floor

Look up

Keep the forearms parallel to the floor

Wheel
All Levels

Wheel requires muscle length and strength; holding it with deep rhythmical breathing is a sign that you are making good progress in your asanas. Relax afterwards on your back with bent knees (see p189).

Beginner

1 Lie on your back with your knees bent and your feet a hip-width apart and flat on the mat. Hold your ankles. Breathe deeply and rhythmically.

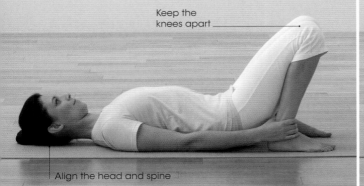

Keep the knees apart

Align the head and spine

2 Keep your head, shoulders, and feet on the floor as you inhale and lift your hips up as high as possible. Hold for a couple of deep, rhythmical breaths, then continue with Step 3 or lower your hips back to the floor and relax.

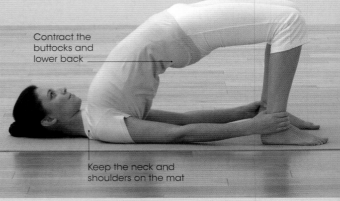

Contract the buttocks and lower back

Keep the neck and shoulders on the mat

Intermediate and Advanced

3 Still breathing deeply and rhythmically, continue lifting your hips and take your hands next to your ears, with your fingers facing your shoulders. Keep your feet parallel to each other.

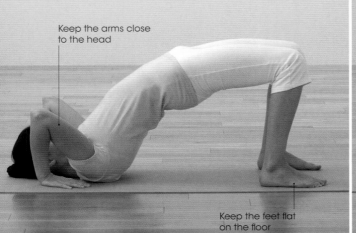

Keep the arms close to the head

Keep the feet flat on the floor

4 Inhale, push on your hands, lift your head, and gently place the top of your head on the floor. Your elbows should be pointing backwards and your arms bent.

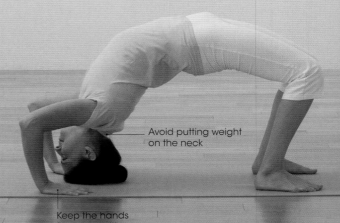

Avoid putting weight on the neck

Keep the hands firmly in position

5 To come into the full pose, on the next inhalation, straighten your arms to lift your torso. If you find it difficult to straighten your arms, try balancing on your toes; then, once your arms are straight, lower your heels. Hold for a few breaths, then come out of the pose by bending your arms and following Steps 3, 2, and 1 in that order. Make sure you release the pose before it becomes too tiring, so you have the strength to lower your neck safely back to the floor. Repeat this sequence 1–2 more times.

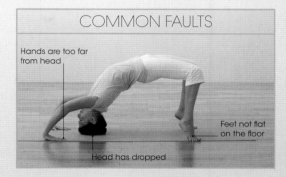

COMMON FAULTS

Hands are too far from head

Feet not flat on the floor

Head has dropped

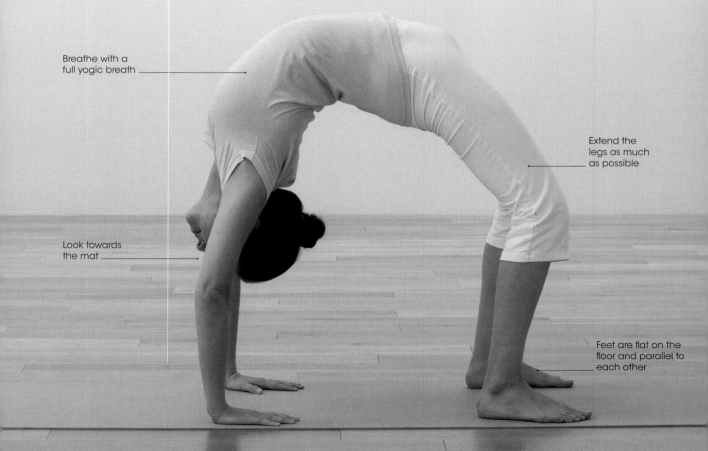

Breathe with a full yogic breath

Extend the legs as much as possible

Look towards the mat

Feet are flat on the floor and parallel to each other

Wheel
Variations

These advanced Wheel variations are best practised with another person or a teacher standing next to you, ready to hold your hips in case you start falling to one side.

Start with

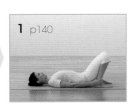

1 p140

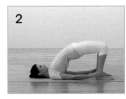

2

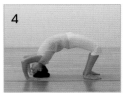

3

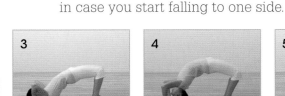

4

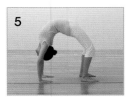

5

One Leg Up
Advanced

Starting from Wheel Step 5, shift your weight to your right leg. On an inhalation, lift your left leg. Hold your breath, then lower the leg back to the floor on an exhalation. Repeat on the other side, then either continue with One Arm Up (see right) or come out of the pose by bending your arms and repeating Wheel Steps 3, 2, and 1 in that order.

Stretch the toes

Keep the knees straight

One Arm Up
Advanced

Starting from Wheel Step 5, shift your weight to your left arm. Inhale and lift your right arm, then place your right hand on your right thigh, fingers turned inwards. Hold your breath for a few seconds, then, on an exhalation, lower your right arm back to the floor. Repeat on the other side, then come out of the pose by bending your arms and repeating Wheel Steps 3, 2, and 1 in that order.

Keep the hips level

Keep the legs apart

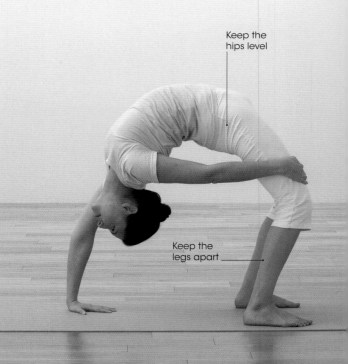

Full Wheel from Standing
Advanced

1 Stand near the front of the mat with your legs 50cm (20in) apart and your feet turned slightly outwards. Hold your hands in Prayer Position (see p50) in front of your chest.

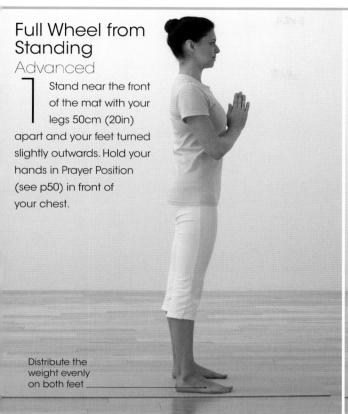

Distribute the weight evenly on both feet

2 Inhale and lift your arms over your head. Drop your head back and start bending backwards, holding your arms out straight behind you.

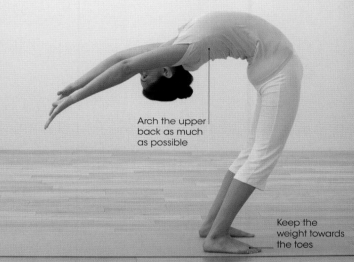

Arch the upper back as much as possible

Keep the weight towards the toes

3 Bend your knees slightly and continue bending backwards, taking your extended arms closer to the floor. Hold your breath and keep your balance by shifting your body weight as far forwards as possible.

Keep the arms straight

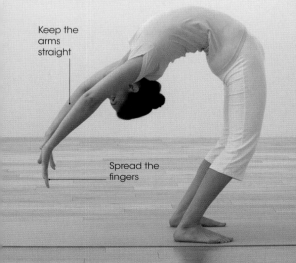

Spread the fingers

4 Once you are near the floor, let your body weight shift gently towards your arms. As soon as your hands meet the floor, bend your elbows slightly to protect your wrists. Take a few breaths, then return to Step 1 by inhaling and quickly shifting your weight to the front. Alternatively, bend your elbows and come up by following Wheel Steps 3, 2, and 1, in that order.

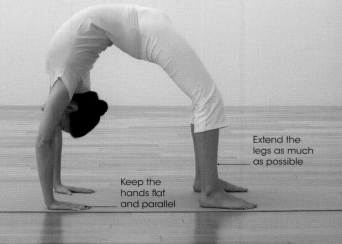

Extend the legs as much as possible

Keep the hands flat and parallel

9 Half Spinal Twist
Ardha Matsyendrasana

Lateral rotation is very important for achieving complete flexibility of the spine. These various twisting asanas work on the rotation of all the vertebrae, as well as on rotation of the hip joint. You should follow each of them with Child's Pose (see p191) as a relaxing counterpose. This asana is named after the great yogic sage, Matsyendranath.

BENEFITS

PHYSICAL
• Helps to improve the flexibility of the spine.
• Helps to tone the roots of the spinal nerves.
• Helps to energize the gastrointestinal system.
• Enhances the functioning of the large intestine.
• Improves the appetite.

MENTAL
• Rotation or twisting of the spine is not a common movement in daily life. By exploring this unusual movement, your mind will also become more flexible and adaptable.

Half Spinal Twist
Beginner

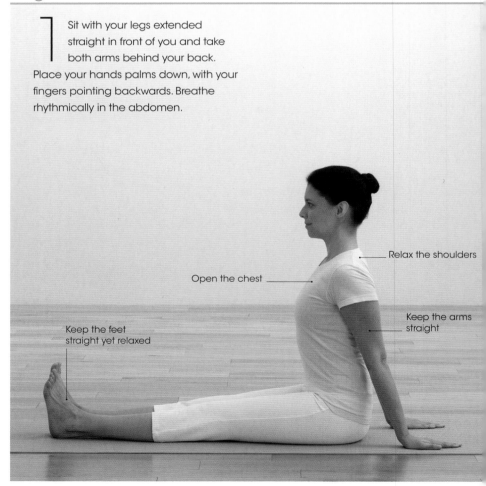

1 Sit with your legs extended straight in front of you and take both arms behind your back. Place your hands palms down, with your fingers pointing backwards. Breathe rhythmically in the abdomen.

Relax the shoulders

Open the chest

Keep the arms straight

Keep the feet straight yet relaxed

2 Place your left foot flat on the mat outside your right calf. Inhale and lift your right arm straight up.

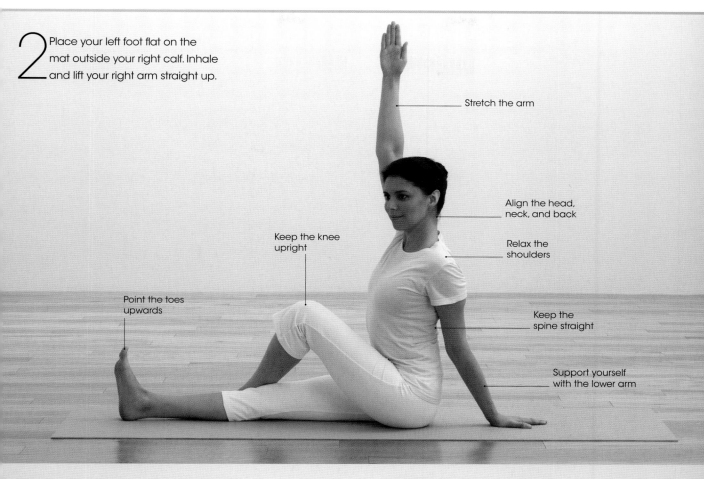

Stretch the arm

Align the head, neck, and back

Relax the shoulders

Keep the knee upright

Keep the spine straight

Point the toes upwards

Support yourself with the lower arm

3 To come into the full pose, exhale, bring your right arm down and push it against the outside of your left leg. Catch hold of the sole of your left foot or ankle. Turn your chest, head, and eyes to the left. Breathe slowly in your abdomen. Hold for up to 1 minute. Slowly release first your head, then your spine. Repeat on the other side.

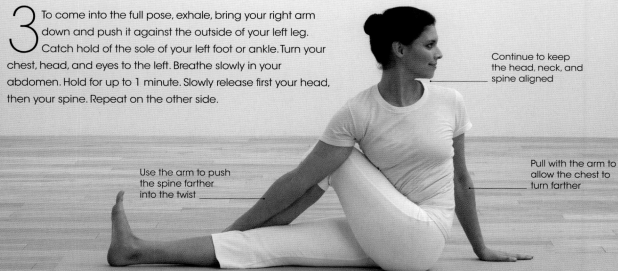

Continue to keep the head, neck, and spine aligned

Pull with the arm to allow the chest to turn farther

Use the arm to push the spine farther into the twist

Half Spinal Twist
Intermediate and Advanced

The lumbar area does not twist easily, so you need to rotate the cervical and thoracic areas of your spine. Keeping your chest open and your neck straight is the best basis for a good twist.

1 Start by sitting on your heels and placing your palms face down on your thighs.

2 Keeping with your palms on your thighs, adjust yourself so you are sitting to the right of your feet, with your buttocks evenly on the floor.

Keep the back, neck, and head aligned

Keep the spine erect and aligned

3 Take your left foot over your right thigh, placing it flat on the mat close to your knee. Support your body with your left arm behind your back. Inhale and lift your right arm straight up.

4 To come into the full pose, exhale, bring your right arm down, and push it against the outside of your left knee as you try to catch hold of the sole of your left foot or your left ankle. Turn your chest, head, and eyes to the left. Breathe slowly in your abdomen. Hold the pose for up to one minute. Slowly release first your head, then your spine. Repeat on the other side, then either practise the variations (see pp148–9) or relax.

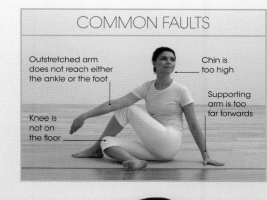

COMMON FAULTS

Outstretched arm does not reach either the ankle or the foot

Chin is too high

Supporting arm is too far forwards

Knee is not on the floor

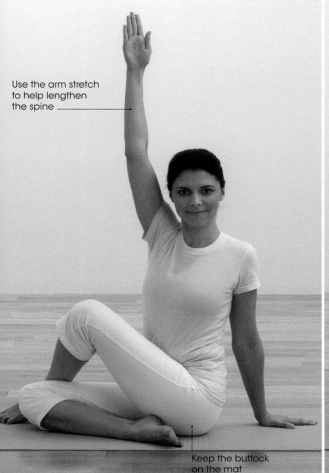

Use the arm stretch to help lengthen the spine

Keep the buttock on the mat

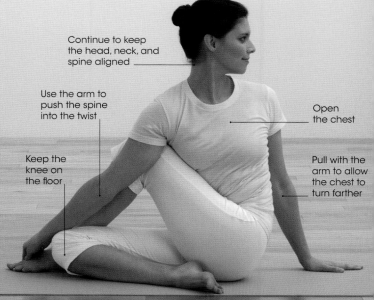

Continue to keep the head, neck, and spine aligned

Use the arm to push the spine into the twist

Keep the knee on the floor

Open the chest

Pull with the arm to allow the chest to turn farther

Half Spinal Twist
Variations

These variations increase both the rotation of the spine and the stretch in the abductor muscles on the outside of your thighs. Only practise them if you can keep your back, neck, and head upright.

Start with

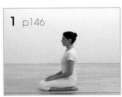

1 p146

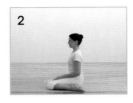

2

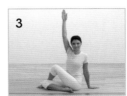

3

Wrist Grasp
Advanced

Starting from Intermediate Half Spinal Twist Step 3, take your right arm through the space between your left knee and your right leg. Hold your left hand or wrist. Hold with slow abdominal breathing for up to 2 minutes. Repeat on the other side.

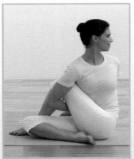

Front view This view shows clearly the full opening of the chest in the pose.

Ankle Clasp
Advanced

Starting from Wrist Grasp (see left), take your left foot closer to your hip. Place your left arm against your back, and try to hold your left ankle. Hold your right knee with your right hand and use your right arm as a lever to help you to twist to the left. Breathe slowly and hold for up to 2 minutes. Repeat on the other side.

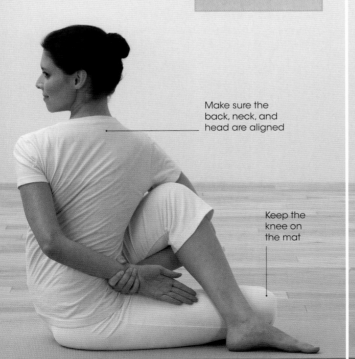

Make sure the back, neck, and head are aligned

Keep the knee on the mat

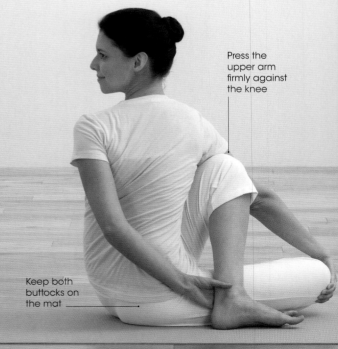

Press the upper arm firmly against the knee

Keep both buttocks on the mat

Start with

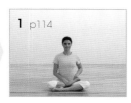

1 p114

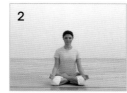

2

Full Spinal Twist
Advanced

This is Purna Matsyendrasana or Full Spinal Twist.
Starting from Lotus Step 2, lift your left leg and
catch hold of your left foot with your right hand.
Keep your left arm behind your back. Turn your
head to the left and look over your left shoulder.
Hold for up to 1 minute with rhythmical
breathing. Slowly release first your head, then
your spine. Repeat on the other side.

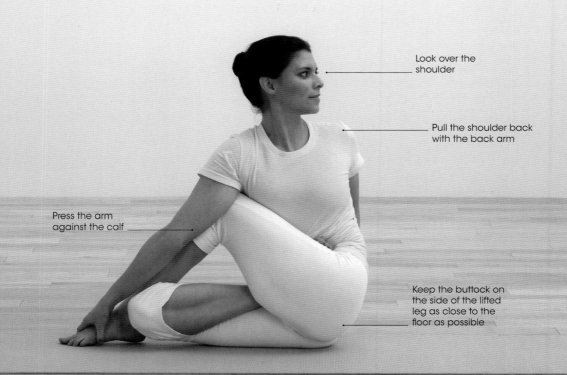

Look over the
shoulder

Pull the shoulder back
with the back arm

Press the arm
against the calf

Keep the buttock on
the side of the lifted
leg as close to the
floor as possible

10a Crow
Kakasana

Strengthening the arms and the shoulder girdle is a main concern in any physical exercise programme. Instead of using weights, the Yogis developed balancing asanas such as Crow and its variations. In these, the body weight shifts from the feet, legs, and hips to the hands, arms, and shoulders. Relax afterwards in Child's Pose (see p191).

BENEFITS

PHYSICAL
- Helps to develop strength and flexibility in the wrists.
- Strengthens the tricep muscles.
- Strengthens the shoulder muscles.
- The variations further strengthen the muscles of the legs, hips, and back.

MENTAL
- When you are practising this pose, you have to evaluate how much of your body weight you can place on your arms and hands. If you place too little weight on them, you will not be able to lift your feet off the floor. After a period of testing and hesitation, one concentrated, determined movement will lift you into the pose. Crow therefore helps to develop your determination as well as your powers of concentration.

Crow
Beginner

1 Sit in a squatting position with your legs and feet apart. Taking your shoulders in front of your knees, place your palms on the mat in front of you. Keep your arms slightly bent and adopt the correct position for your hands and elbows (see inset). Breathe slowly and rhythmically.

Hand and Elbow Position
Spread your fingers wide apart, turn your wrists inwards, and bend your elbows outwards.

Knees are wide apart

Look straight ahead

2 Come up onto your toes, lifting your hips, and keeping your knees pressed firmly against your upper arms. Continue breathing rhythmically in the abdomen.

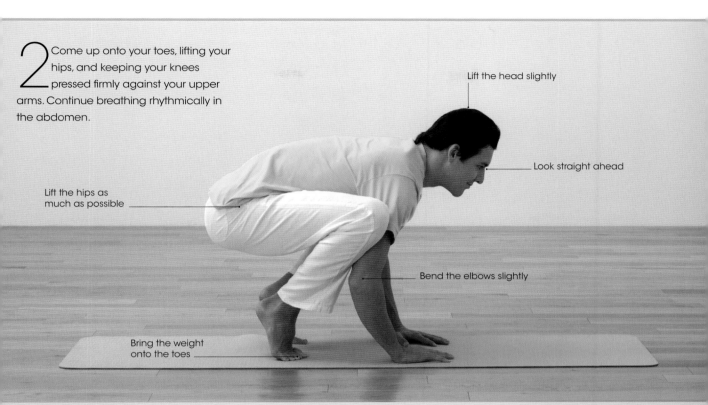

Lift the head slightly

Look straight ahead

Lift the hips as much as possible

Bend the elbows slightly

Bring the weight onto the toes

3 Breathing more deeply, focus on a point in front of you, then slowly move forwards, shifting your weight away from your feet and onto your wrists. Your elbows should be slightly bent and your knees resting on your upper arms. Continue with Step 4 (see p152) or hold for a few moments, then exhale and return to a squatting position.

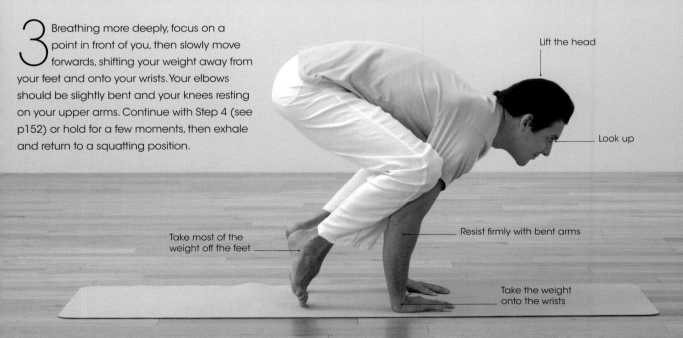

Lift the head

Look up

Take most of the weight off the feet

Resist firmly with bent arms

Take the weight onto the wrists

Crow
Intermediate and Advanced

Side Crow (see right) is far simpler to perform than it looks. What you need is a very steady base to support the weight of your legs. Side Crow also helps to develop lateral balancing.

Start with

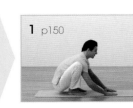
1 p150

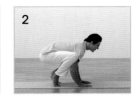
2

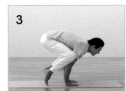
3

4 If your wrists are strong enough, come into the full pose. Starting from Crow Step 3, inhale, hold your breath, then slowly move your weight farther forwards until your feet lift off the floor. Balance for a few moments, then exhale, and return to Step 2. Once you can achieve the full pose, hold it as you breathe rhythmically for up to 30 seconds.

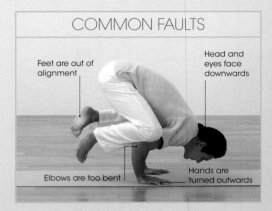

COMMON FAULTS

Feet are out of alignment

Head and eyes face downwards

Elbows are too bent

Hands are turned outwards

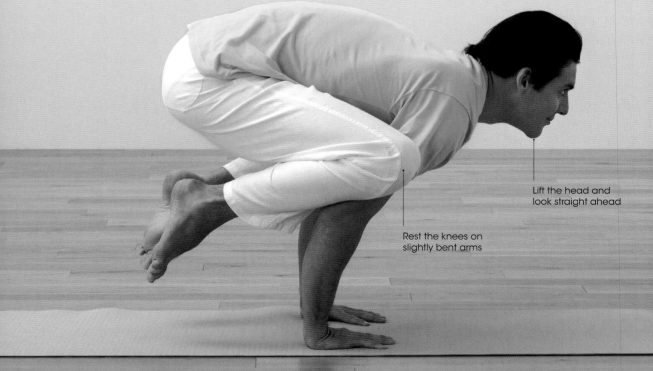

Lift the head and look straight ahead

Rest the knees on slightly bent arms

Side Crow
Advanced Variation

1 Starting from a kneeling squat, place both hands flat on the floor, 50cm (20in) apart, to the right of your legs. Walk both feet to the left.

2 Make sure your feet are 50cm (20in) from your left hand and in line with your hands. Bend your knees and take your legs onto the top of your left elbow, inhale and hold your breath as you shift your weight forwards until your feet come off the floor.

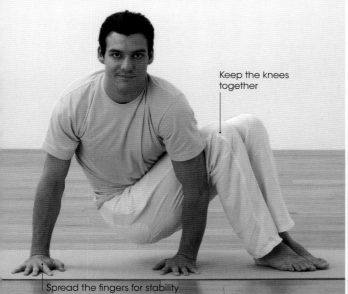

Keep the knees together

Spread the fingers for stability

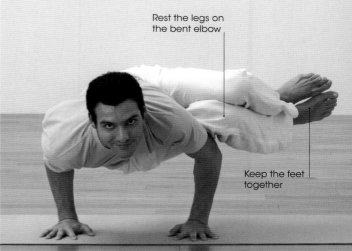

Rest the legs on the bent elbow

Keep the feet together

3 Breathing deeply and rhythmically, shift the weight of your head, torso, feet, and legs forwards as you slowly extend your legs. Hold for as long as deep rhythmical breathing allows you, then bend your knees and come back to a kneeling squat. Repeat on the other side.

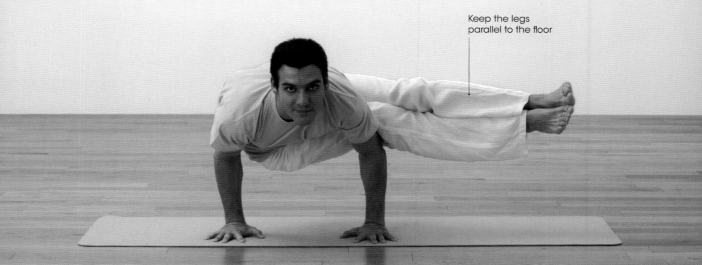

Keep the legs parallel to the floor

10b Peacock
Mayurasana

When you are practising this pose, your body resembles a peacock with its feathers spread out behind. It is an excellent balancing exercise. In addition, with just a few seconds' work, you will have strengthened many of the muscles in your body and will have toned your lungs and abdominal organs. Relax afterwards in Child's Pose (see p191).

BENEFITS

PHYSICAL
- Strengthens the muscles of the legs, arms, back, abdomen, shoulders, and neck.
- Tones the lungs.
- Tones the abdominal organs.
- Helps to overcome constipation.
- Gives the whole body a powerful tonic.

MENTAL
- The strong muscular effort, deep breathing, and keen concentration required for this pose help to overcome sluggishness (tamas; see p212) as well as hyperactivity (rajas; see p212).

Peacock
Beginner

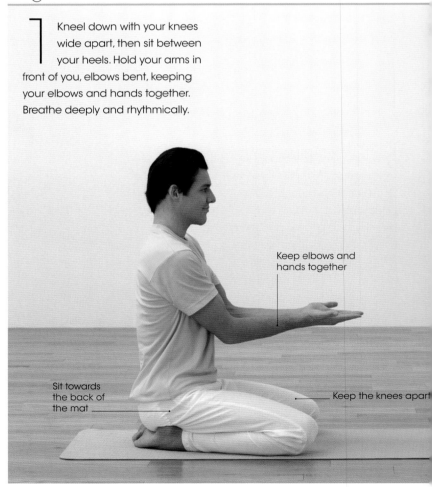

1 Kneel down with your knees wide apart, then sit between your heels. Hold your arms in front of you, elbows bent, keeping your elbows and hands together. Breathe deeply and rhythmically.

Keep elbows and hands together

Sit towards the back of the mat

Keep the knees apart

2 Lean forwards, lifting your hips and placing your palms on the mat close to your knees, fingers pointing backwards. Keeping your elbows together, place your upper abdomen against them. For some women this may be difficult, in which case, keep your elbows farther apart.

Keep the head lifted

Rest the abdomen on the elbows

3 Slowly lean forwards and lower your forehead to the floor. Keep your abdomen pressed tightly against your elbows and continue breathing rhythmically.

Keep the elbows together

Keep the feet together

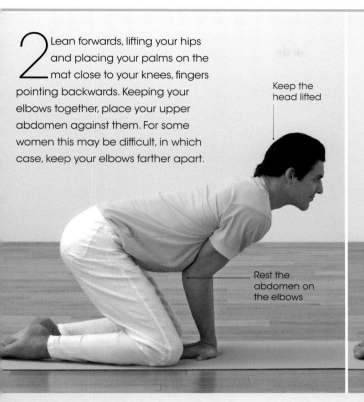

4 Stretch one leg out, and then the other. Tuck your toes under. Resist the pressure of your elbows with your abdominal muscles. Continue with Step 5 (see p156) or come down by exhaling, then lowering your feet and knees to the floor. Sit up and shake out your wrists.

Stay strong in the arms

Keep the knees straight

Place the forehead on the mat

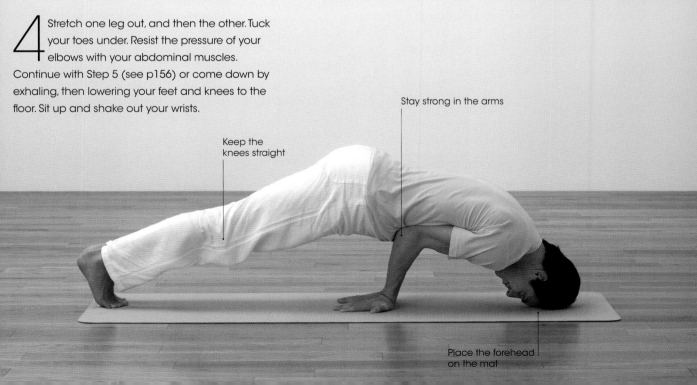

Peacock
Intermediate and Advanced

Each asana acts on specific pressure points of the body, allowing the release of pent-up prana, or vital energy (see p178). Peacock helps prana to circulate from the solar plexus throughout the whole body.

Start with

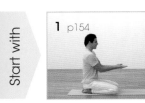

1 p154

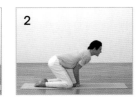

2

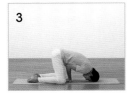

3

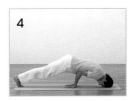

4

Intermediate

5 Starting from Peacock Step 4, on an inhalation, lift your head and chest. Take one more deep breath and prepare to contract the muscles of your legs, back, abdomen, and neck. Continue with Step 6 or come down by exhaling and lowering your feet and knees to the floor. Sit up and shake out your wrists.

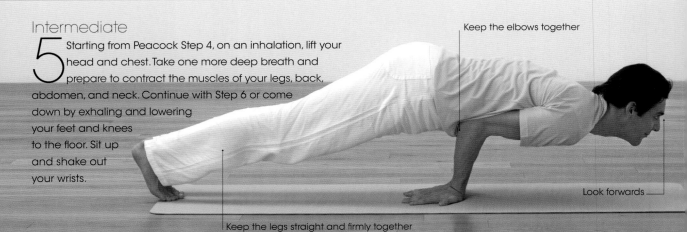

Keep the elbows together

Look forwards

Keep the legs straight and firmly together

Advanced

6 To come into the final pose, after the deepest possible inhalation, hold your breath, make your body stiff, and tiptoe forwards until your legs come off the floor. Exhale, then lower your feet and knees to the floor. Sit up and shake out your wrists.

COMMON FAULTS

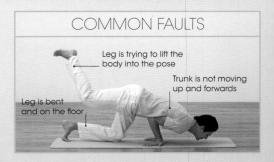

Leg is trying to lift the body into the pose

Trunk is not moving up and forwards

Leg is bent and on the floor

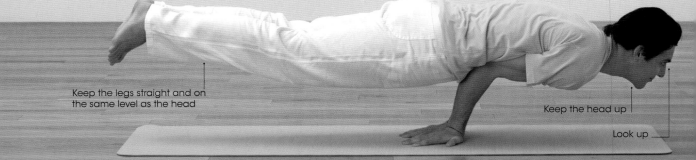

Keep the legs straight and on the same level as the head

Keep the head up

Look up

Head to Floor
Advanced Variation

Starting from Peacock Step 6 (see opposite), continue shifting your weight forwards until your forehead touches the mat and your legs come high off the floor. Try to hold for 3 breaths, then release. Exhale, then lower your feet and knees to the floor. Sit up and shake out your wrists.

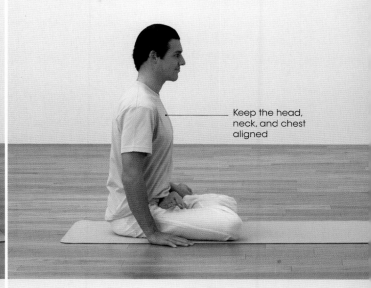

Keep the legs, hips, and spine aligned

Lotus Peacock
Advanced Variation

1 Sit cross-legged; come into Lotus (see p114) by lifting your left foot onto the top of your right thigh, then your right foot onto the top of your left thigh.

Keep the head, neck, and chest aligned

2 Move your body forwards until you are balancing on your knees. Place your palms flat, with your fingers pointing towards your legs.

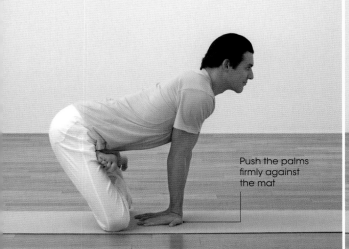

Push the palms firmly against the mat

3 Bend your elbows and place them against your abdomen. Inhale and move your body forwards, lifting your head and chest together with your bent legs. Hold for up to 3 breaths, then come down by following Steps 2 and 1 in that order. Repeat with your legs crossed the other way.

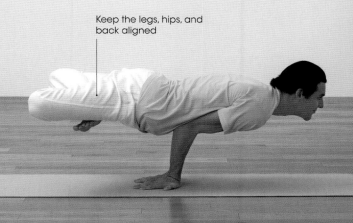

Keep the legs, hips, and back aligned

Standing Balances
All Levels

Standing on one leg demands concentration and single-mindedness rather than physical prowess. To help you find your point of balance, alternate your weight between your heel and toes.

Tree
Beginner

1 Stand up straight, focusing on a spot in front of you for balance. Breathe slowly from your abdomen. Lift your left foot and place it against your right thigh. Point your left knee outwards.

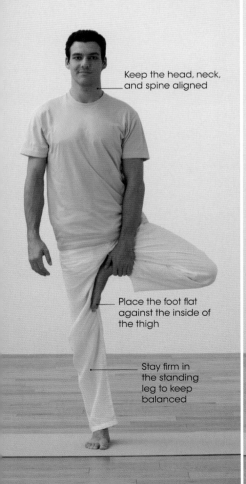

Keep the head, neck, and spine aligned

Place the foot flat against the inside of the thigh

Stay firm in the standing leg to keep balanced

2 When you feel secure in your balance, release the hold on your foot and place your hands in Prayer Position (see p50) in front of your chest. Keep up the rhythmical breathing.

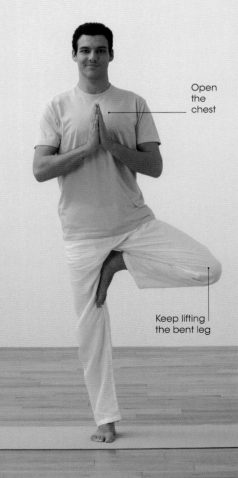

Open the chest

Keep lifting the bent leg

3 With an inhalation, slowly lift your arms. Hold the pose for up to 1 minute. Release, then repeat on the other side. Practise another standing asana (see pp159–69) or go directly to final relaxation (see pp192–3).

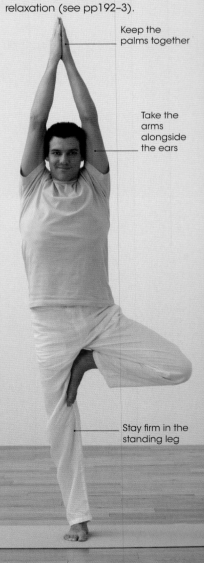

Keep the palms together

Take the arms alongside the ears

Stay firm in the standing leg

Half Lotus Tree
Intermediate Variation

1 Stand up straight, focusing on a spot in front of you to help you keep your balance. Lift your left foot and place it on top of your right thigh in Half Lotus. Release your hold on your foot and take your arms alongside your body. Press firmly into the foot of the standing leg.

2 Slowly lift your arms. Hold for up to 1 minute, breathing rhythmically, then release and repeat on the other side. Practise another standing asana (see pp159–69) or go directly to final relaxation (see pp192–3).

Eagle
Intermediate

Stand with both knees slightly bent. Place your right knee on top of your left knee and lock your left foot behind your right calf. Place your left upper arm inside your right elbow and bring your palms together in front of your face. Hold for up to 30 seconds, breathing rhythmically. Release and repeat on the other side. Practise another standing asana (see pp160–69) or go directly to final relaxation (see pp192–3).

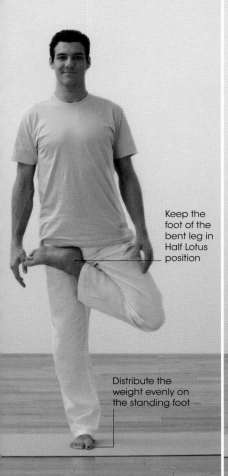

Keep the foot of the bent leg in Half Lotus position

Distribute the weight evenly on the standing foot

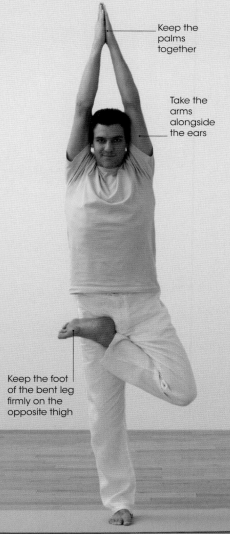

Keep the palms together

Take the arms alongside the ears

Keep the foot of the bent leg firmly on the opposite thigh

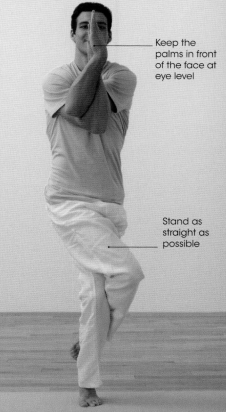

Keep the palms in front of the face at eye level

Stand as straight as possible

Dancing Lord Siva
All Levels

Focusing on the vertical position of the leg and arm on one side of the body creates a stable base. Then you can easily develop the backward bending movement on the other side of the body.

Beginner and Intermediate

1 Stand firmly on both feet. Balance on your left foot, lift your right ankle, and grasp it with your right hand. Establish your balance by breathing slowly and rhythmically.

2 With an inhalation, stretch your left arm up, taking it alongside your left ear. Extend your elbow and stretch your fingers upwards. Look firmly at a point in front of you, breathe slowly and rhythmically, and affirm your balance on your left foot.

3 Push your right foot backwards as you lean slightly forwards with your upper body. Breathe deeply and rhythmically. Hold for up to 30 seconds, then release and repeat on the other side. Continue with Step 4 (see opposite), or practise Standing Forward Bend (see pp162–3) or Triangle (see pp164–9), or go directly to final relaxation (see pp192–3).

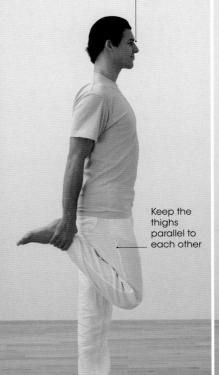

Concentrate on a spot in front of you

Keep the thighs parallel to each other

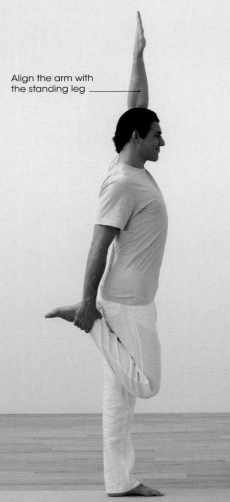

Align the arm with the standing leg

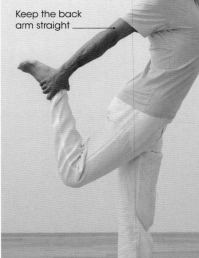

Keep the arm vertical and alongside the ear

Keep the back arm straight

Keep the weight firmly on the standing foot

Advanced

4 Starting from Dancing Lord Siva Step 3, pull your right foot close to your right shoulder until you can lift your elbow. Rotate your wrist so you are holding the upper part of your foot. Breathe deeply and rhythmically. Hold for up to 30 seconds, then release and repeat on the other side.

5 To come into the full pose, bring your left arm over your head and lower your left hand to place it on your right foot so that you are holding your foot with both hands. Hold the pose for up to 30 seconds, breathing deeply and rhythmically. Release and repeat on the other side. Practise Standing Forward Bend (see pp162–3) or Triangle (see pp164–9), or go directly to final relaxation (see pp192–3).

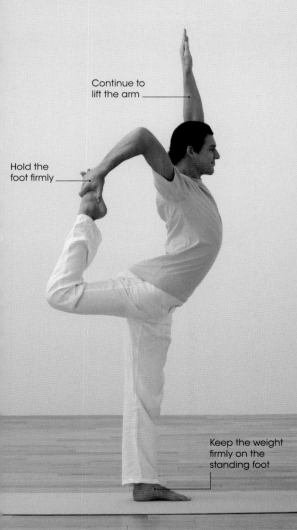

Continue to lift the arm

Hold the foot firmly

Keep the weight firmly on the standing foot

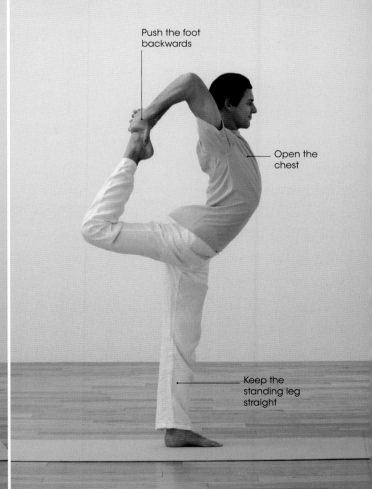

Push the foot backwards

Open the chest

Keep the standing leg straight

11 Standing Forward Bend
Pada Hasthasana.

If you notice that your legs are stiff from too much sitting on chairs, practise this Standing Forward Bend. Using the pull of gravity, this pose quickly lengthens the muscles and ligaments of the entire posterior face of your body – from your heels to the middle of your back. It also prepares you for the next asana, Triangle (see pp164–9).

BENEFITS

PHYSICAL
- Lengthens the muscles in the legs, hips, and lower back.
- Moderately increases the blood supply to the brain.
- Progressively trims the waist when accompanied by proper diet.
- Helps to overcome constipation.

MENTAL
- The stimulation of the spine, the activated sense of balance, and the extra blood supply to the brain produced by this pose all bring relief from tamas, a state of low energy characterized by sluggishness, inertia, sleepiness, forgetfulness, and depression (see p212).

CAUTION If the backs of your knees are over-extended, you should focus on keeping your knees straight without pushing them backwards.

Standing Forward Bend
All Levels

Beginner and Intermediate

1 Stand upright, with your legs together. Inhale and stretch your arms up alongside your ears.

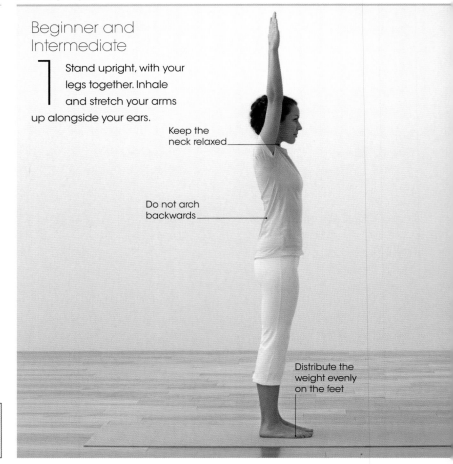

Keep the neck relaxed

Do not arch backwards

Distribute the weight evenly on the feet

2 Exhale and bend forwards from the hips so that you make a horizontal line with your arms and upper body.

Keep the back, head, and arms aligned

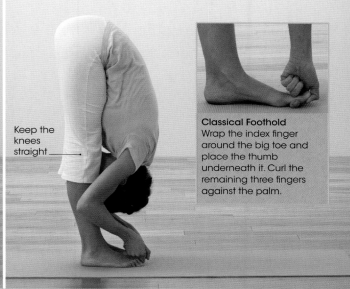

Distribute the weight evenly on the feet

3 Continue exhaling and bending forwards. Catch hold of your ankles or calves, or hold onto your big toes in the Classical Foothold (see below). Hold for up to 1 minute with slow rhythmical breathing. Continue with Step 4 or inhale and come back up, with your arms and head hanging, then return to standing.

Keep the knees straight

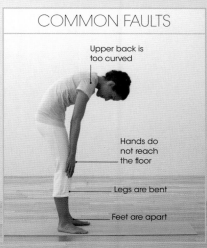

Classical Foothold
Wrap the index finger around the big toe and place the thumb underneath it. Curl the remaining three fingers against the palm.

Advanced

4 If you can hold your toes, come into the full pose by bringing your arms behind your knees and holding your elbows. With an exhalation, push your arms down along your calves. Alternatively, for a greater stretch in the legs, slide the palms of your hands under your feet (see below). Hold either position for up to 1 minute, with slow rhythmical breathing, then come back up as in Step 3.

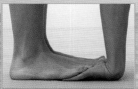

Alternative Foothold Slide the palms under the feet.

Increase the stretch in the spine by pushing the arms farther down

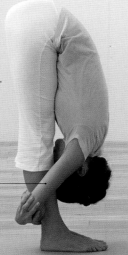

COMMON FAULTS

Upper back is too curved

Hands do not reach the floor

Legs are bent

Feet are apart

12 Triangle
Trikonasana

Triangle is a unique asana. Its lateral bend stretches and strengthens several muscles on the side of the body at the same time. It also helps with balance. It is the last of the twelve basic asanas in the cycle. After you have practised Triangle, end your session with final relaxation (see pp192–3) in order to reap all the benefits of your practice.

BENEFITS

PHYSICAL
• Increases the sideways mobility of the lumbar and thoracic areas of the spine.
• Strengthens and lengthens the muscles of the legs and back.
• Tones the spinal nerves.
• Tones the abdominal organs.
• Improves the movement of food through the intestines and so invigorates the appetite.

MENTAL
• Working the muscles of the legs and back while still breathing calmly in the abdomen and consciously trying to relax presents both a physical and a mental challenge. Triangle can teach you how to face a challenging task while staying mentally calm and detached.
• Strengthens concentration and mental determination.

Triangle
All Levels

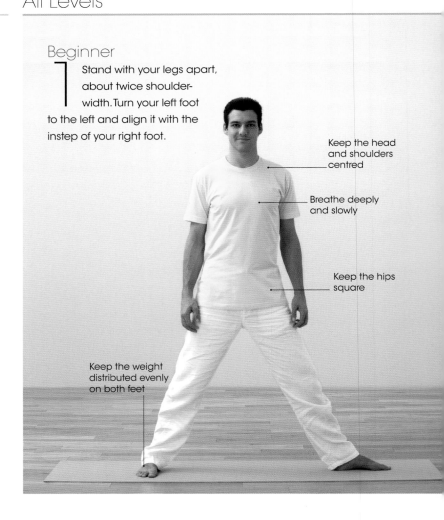

Beginner
1 Stand with your legs apart, about twice shoulder-width. Turn your left foot to the left and align it with the instep of your right foot.

Keep the head and shoulders centred

Breathe deeply and slowly

Keep the hips square

Keep the weight distributed evenly on both feet

2 Inhale and take your right arm up alongside your right ear.

Focus on the stretch from the foot to the raised hand

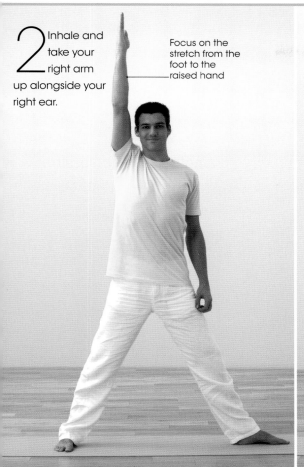

3 If you are unable to reach over your head without bending your leg (see Step 3, below), exhale and bend your trunk to the left. Bend your left leg, and place your left hand on your left foot. Hold for up to one minute, then repeat on the other side.

Align the hips, trunk, and arm in one horizontal line

Look up

Turn the face forwards

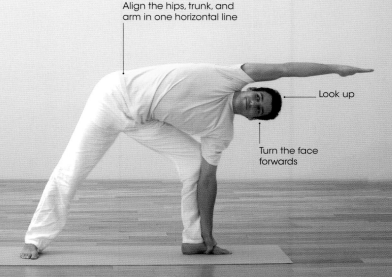

Intermediate and Advanced

3 If you are able to reach over your head without bending your leg, come into the full pose from Step 2. Exhale and bend to the left, keeping your left knee straight. Catch hold of your ankle or your calf. Hold for up to one minute, then repeat on the other side.

Do not lean on the lower hand

Keep some weight on the back foot

COMMON FAULTS

Upper arm is bent

Head not in line with the spine

Eyes are looking down

Front foot is not aligned with back foot

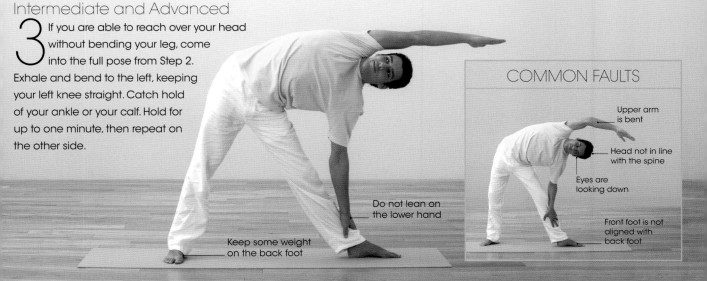

Triangle
Variations

These variations add first a hip rotation and then a spinal twist to the lateral bend that you do when you practise Triangle. This combination of movements gives your back a complete workout.

Simple Hip Twist
Beginner

1 Stand with your legs about twice shoulder-width apart. Turn your left foot to the left and your right foot slightly in. Interlock your fingers behind your back. Inhale deeply.

2 With an exhalation, bend your body over your left leg, bringing your forehead to your left knee. Breathe rhythmically, holding for up to 1 minute, then repeat on the other side.

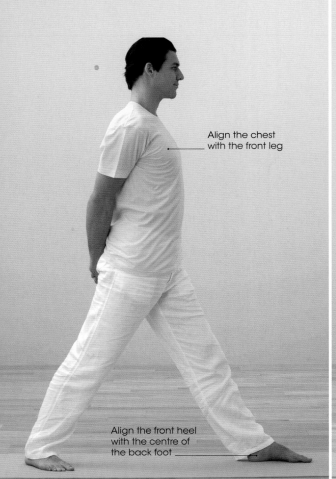

Align the chest with the front leg

Align the front heel with the centre of the back foot

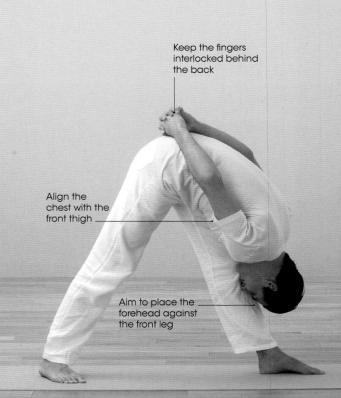

Keep the fingers interlocked behind the back

Align the chest with the front thigh

Aim to place the forehead against the front leg

Triangle with Spinal Twist
Intermediate

1 Stand with your legs about twice shoulder-width apart. Turn your right foot to the right and your left foot slightly in. Lift your arms parallel to the floor and twist your body as far as possible to the right. Inhale deeply.

2 With an exhalation, twist and bend your body from the waist. Place your left hand either on top of your right ankle or flat on the floor outside your right foot. Raise your right arm straight upwards and look up at it. Breathe rhythmically, holding for up to 1 minute, then repeat on the other side.

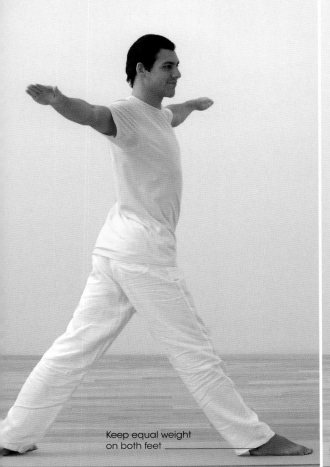

Keep equal weight on both feet

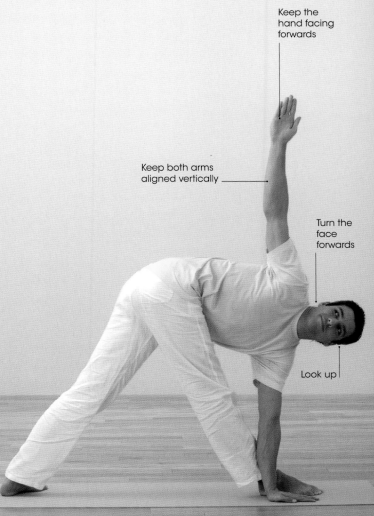

Keep the hand facing forwards

Keep both arms aligned vertically

Turn the face forwards

Look up

Triangle
Variations (continued)

These variations give special attention to stretching and strengthening the pelvic girdle. The isometric contraction of the quadriceps muscles provides an intense workout for the thighs.

Triangle with Bent Knee
Intermediate

1 Stand with your legs farther apart than in Triangle Step 1 (see p164). Turn your left foot to the left, bend your left knee, and rest your left forearm on it. Keep your right leg straight. Breathe rhythmically.

Lower your hips as much as possible

2 Turn your torso to the left, exhale, and place both palms on the floor, parallel to each other, and to the inside of your left foot.

Keep the extended leg straight

Keep the back foot flat on the floor

3 Inhale and lift your right arm, taking it alongside your right ear. Hold for up to 30 seconds, breathing rhythmically. To come out of the pose, lift your left arm straight up and, with a push of your left leg, stand up straight again. Repeat on the other side.

Turn the face forwards

Look up

Keep the left calf vertical

Keep the back foot flat on the floor

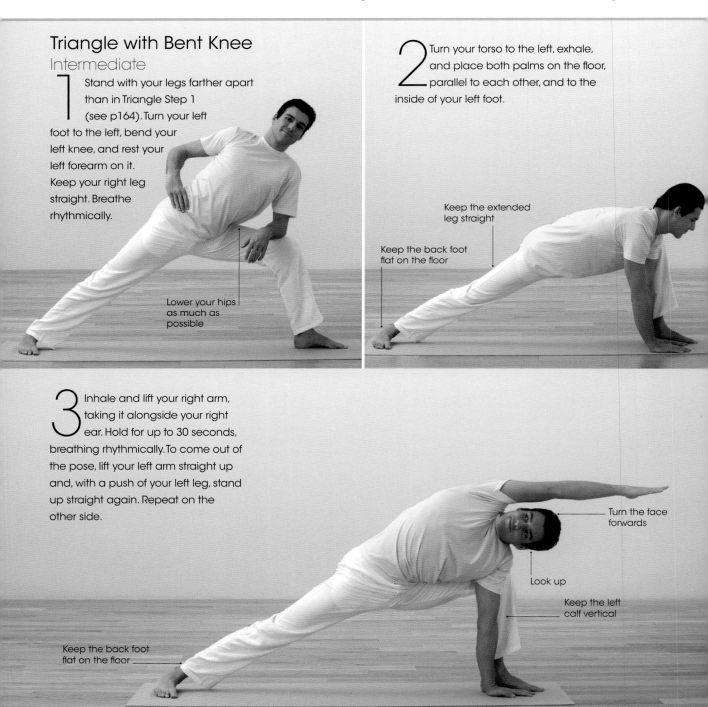

Head to Toe
Advanced

4 Starting from Triangle with Bent Knee Step 2 (see opposite), take your hands behind your back and interlock your fingers. Inhale and lift your back until it is aligned with your left leg, keeping your balance on both feet.

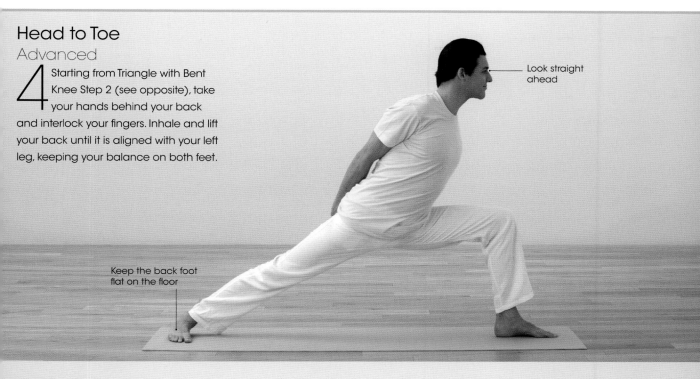

Look straight ahead

Keep the back foot flat on the floor

5 Exhale, bend forwards, and try to place the top of your head on the floor next to your left foot. Hold for up to 30 seconds. With an inhalation, come out of the pose by lifting your torso, then repeat on the other side.

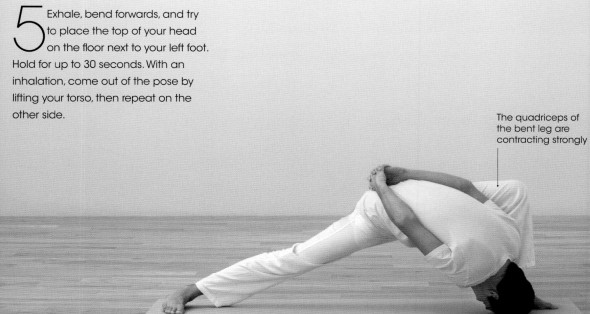

The quadriceps of the bent leg are contracting strongly

Sequences

The sequences in this section offer routines suitable for beginner, intermediate, and advanced levels; at each level there is a 20-, 40-, and 60-minute sequence. Remember to always rest in Corpse Pose (see p46) before you begin.

Beginner's sequences

KEY: CORPSE POSE/CHILD'S POSE/RELAX ON FRONT
– Relax in one of these poses after the exercise

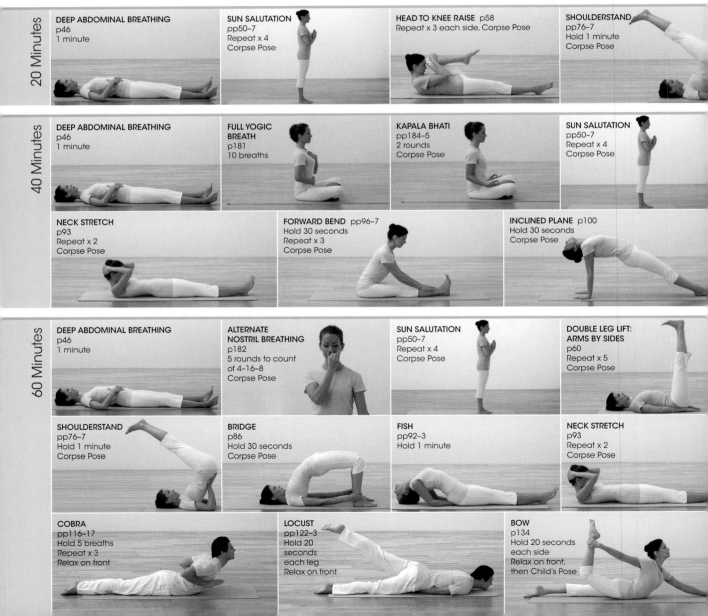

20 Minutes

DEEP ABDOMINAL BREATHING
p46
1 minute

SUN SALUTATION
pp50–7
Repeat x 4
Corpse Pose

HEAD TO KNEE RAISE p58
Repeat x 3 each side, Corpse Pose

SHOULDERSTAND
pp76–7
Hold 1 minute
Corpse Pose

40 Minutes

DEEP ABDOMINAL BREATHING
p46
1 minute

FULL YOGIC
BREATH
p181
10 breaths

KAPALA BHATI
pp184–5
2 rounds
Corpse Pose

SUN SALUTATION
pp50–7
Repeat x 4
Corpse Pose

NECK STRETCH
p93
Repeat x 2
Corpse Pose

FORWARD BEND pp96–7
Hold 30 seconds
Repeat x 3
Corpse Pose

INCLINED PLANE p100
Hold 30 seconds
Corpse Pose

60 Minutes

DEEP ABDOMINAL BREATHING
p46
1 minute

ALTERNATE
NOSTRIL BREATHING
p182
5 rounds to count
of 4–16–8
Corpse Pose

SUN SALUTATION
pp50–7
Repeat x 4
Corpse Pose

DOUBLE LEG LIFT:
ARMS BY SIDES
p60
Repeat x 5
Corpse Pose

SHOULDERSTAND
pp76–7
Hold 1 minute
Corpse Pose

BRIDGE
p86
Hold 30 seconds
Corpse Pose

FISH
pp92–3
Hold 1 minute
Corpse Pose

NECK STRETCH
p93
Repeat x 2
Corpse Pose

COBRA
pp116–17
Hold 5 breaths
Repeat x 3
Relax on front

LOCUST
pp122–3
Hold 20
seconds
each leg
Relax on front

BOW
p134
Hold 20 seconds
each side
Relax on front,
then Child's Pose

Resting Poses

CORPSE POSE p46, 8 breaths between poses, 6-10 minutes in Final relaxation (see pp192-3)
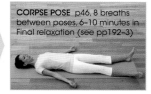

CHILD'S POSE p191
8 breaths after backward bends
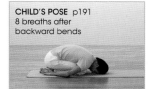

RELAX ON FRONT p190
8 breaths after backward bends
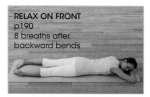

PLOUGH WITH FEET APART p84
Hold 1 minute
Corpse Pose
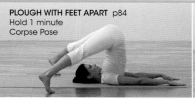

FISH pp92-3
Hold 30 seconds
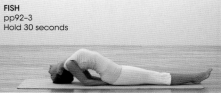

NECK STRETCH p93
Repeat x 2
Final relaxation, about 6 minutes
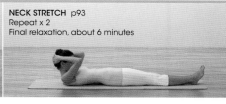

SINGLE LEG LIFT p58
Repeat x 6 each side
Corpse Pose
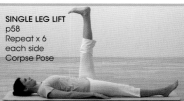

SHOULDERSTAND pp76-7
Hold 1 minute
Corpse Pose
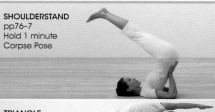

FISH pp92-3
Hold 1 minute
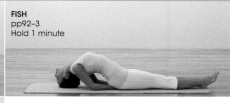

CAMEL p128
Hold up to 30 seconds
Child's Pose
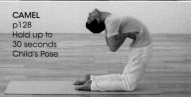

TRIANGLE pp164-5
Hold 20 seconds each side
Corpse Pose
Final Relaxation 10 minutes
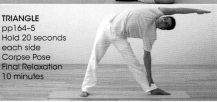

DOLPHIN pp62-3
Repeat x 4
Child's Pose
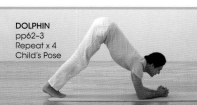

SHOULDERSTAND pp76-7
Hold 1 minute
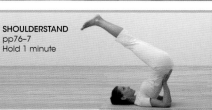

PLOUGH WITH FEET APART p84
Hold 1 minute
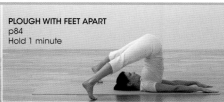

SINGLE LEG FORWARD BEND p102
Hold 1 minute each side

FORWARD BEND pp96-7
Hold 1 minute
Repeat x 2
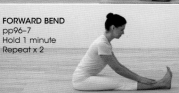

INCLINED PLANE p100
Hold 30 seconds
Corpse Pose
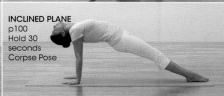

HALF SPINAL TWIST pp144-5
Hold 30 seconds each side
Child's Pose

TREE p158
Hold 20 seconds each side

STANDING FORWARD BEND pp162-3
Hold 1 minute

TRIANGLE pp164-5
Hold 20 seconds each side
Final relaxation 10 minutes

Intermediate sequences

KEY: CORPSE POSE/CHILD'S POSE/RELAX ON FRONT – Relax in one of these poses after the exercise

Resting Poses

CORPSE POSE p46, 8 breaths relaxation between poses, 6–10 minutes Final relaxation (see pp192–3)
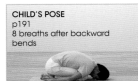

CHILD'S POSE p191 8 breaths after backward bends
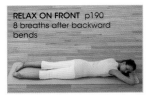

RELAX ON FRONT p190 8 breaths after backward bends

HEADSTAND pp64–7 Hold 1 minute Child's Pose
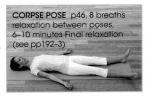

SHOULDERSTAND pp76–8 Hold 1 minute Corpse Pose

FISH pp92–3 Hold 30 seconds

NECK STRETCH p93 Repeat x 2 Corpse Pose

40 Minutes

KAPALA BHATI pp184–5 1 round
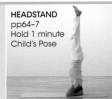

ALTERNATE NOSTRIL BREATHING p182 4 rounds to count of 5-20-10 Corpse Pose
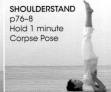

SUN SALUTATION pp50–7 Repeat x 6 Corpse Pose

DEEP STRETCH SINGLE LEG LIFT pp58–9 Hold 30 seconds each side, Corpse Pose
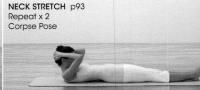

FORWARD BEND: WITH WIDE LEGS p104 Hold 1 minute
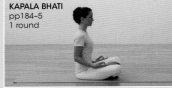

FORWARD BEND pp96–9 Hold 1 minute

INCLINED PLANE p100 Hold 30 seconds
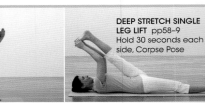

60 Minutes

KAPALA BHATI pp184–5 3 rounds

ALTERNATE NOSTRIL BREATHING pp182 5 rounds count of 5-20-10 Corpse Pose
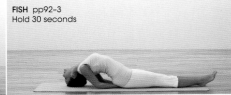

SUN SALUTATION pp50–7 Repeat x 10 Corpse Pose

HEADSTAND: KNEES BENT TO THE SIDES p69 Hold 1 minute Child's Pose

FISH pp92–3 Hold 1 minute Corpse Pose
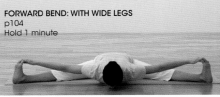

SHOOTING BOW p110 Hold 30 seconds each side
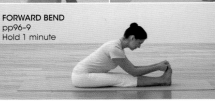

FORWARD BEND pp96–9 Hold 2 minutes
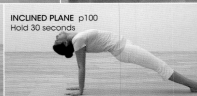

BOW: ROCKING BOW p136 Rock 8 times back and forth Child's Pose
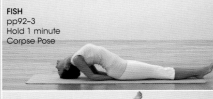

HALF SPINAL TWIST: WRIST GRASP p148 Hold 1 minute each side Child's Pose
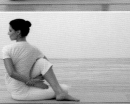

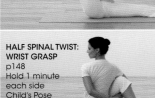

STANDING FORWARD BEND pp162–3 Hold 1 minute
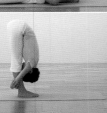
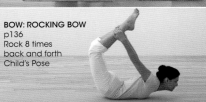
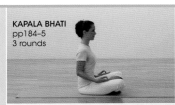

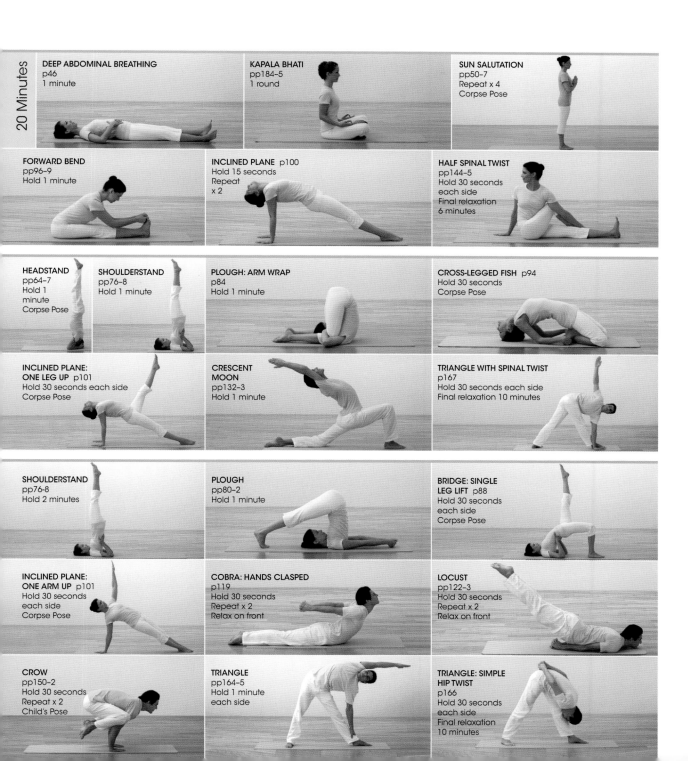

20 Minutes

DEEP ABDOMINAL BREATHING
p46
1 minute

KAPALA BHATI
pp184–5
1 round

SUN SALUTATION
pp50–7
Repeat x 4
Corpse Pose

FORWARD BEND
pp96–9
Hold 1 minute

INCLINED PLANE p100
Hold 15 seconds
Repeat
x 2

HALF SPINAL TWIST
pp144–5
Hold 30 seconds
each side
Final relaxation
6 minutes

HEADSTAND
pp64–7
Hold 1
minute
Corpse Pose

SHOULDERSTAND
pp76–8
Hold 1 minute

PLOUGH: ARM WRAP
p84
Hold 1 minute

CROSS-LEGGED FISH p94
Hold 30 seconds
Corpse Pose

**INCLINED PLANE:
ONE LEG UP** p101
Hold 30 seconds each side
Corpse Pose

**CRESCENT
MOON**
pp132–3
Hold 1 minute

TRIANGLE WITH SPINAL TWIST
p167
Hold 30 seconds each side
Final relaxation 10 minutes

SHOULDERSTAND
pp76–8
Hold 2 minutes

PLOUGH
pp80–2
Hold 1 minute

**BRIDGE: SINGLE
LEG LIFT** p88
Hold 30 seconds
each side
Corpse Pose

**INCLINED PLANE:
ONE ARM UP** p101
Hold 30 seconds
each side
Corpse Pose

COBRA: HANDS CLASPED
p119
Hold 30 seconds
Repeat x 2
Relax on front

LOCUST
pp122–3
Hold 30 seconds
Repeat x 2
Relax on front

CROW
pp150–2
Hold 30 seconds
Repeat x 2
Child's Pose

TRIANGLE
pp164–5
Hold 1 minute
each side

**TRIANGLE: SIMPLE
HIP TWIST**
p166
Hold 30 seconds
each side
Final relaxation
10 minutes

Advanced sequences

KEY: CORPSE POSE/CHILD'S POSE/RELAX ON FRONT – Relax in one of these poses after the exercise

Resting Poses

CORPSE POSE p46, 8 breaths between exercises, 6-10 minutes Final relaxation (see pp192-3)

CHILD'S POSE p191 8 breaths after backward bends

RELAX ON FRONT p190 8 breaths after backward bends

PLOUGH: ARM WRAP p84 Hold 30 seconds

PLOUGH: KNEES BEHIND HEAD p85 Hold 30 seconds

LOTUS FISH p95 Hold 30 seconds Corpse Pose

---

40 Minutes

KAPALA BHATI pp184-5 2 rounds

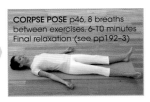

SUN SALUTATION pp50-7 Repeat x 6 Corpse Pose

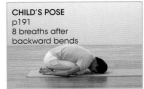

LOTUS HEADSTAND p70 Hold 1 minute

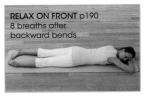

TWISTED LOTUS HEADSTAND p71 Hold 15 seconds each side

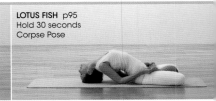

FORWARD BEND pp96-9 Hold 2 minutes Corpse Pose

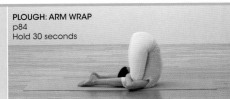

CRESCENT SPLITS p112-13 Hold 30 seconds each side

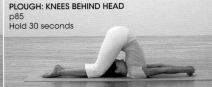

KING COBRA pp120-1 Hold 30 seconds

ROCKING BOW p136 Practise 30 seconds Child's Pose

---

60 Minutes

KAPALA BHATI pp184-5 3 rounds

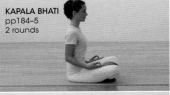

ALTERNATE NOSTRIL BREATHING p182 5 rounds to count of 6-24-12 Corpse Pose

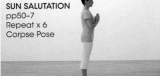

SUN SALUTATION pp50-7 Repeat x 8 Corpse Pose

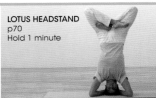

HEADSTAND pp64-7 Hold 3 minutes Child's Pose

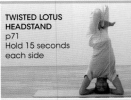

LOTUS FISH p95 Hold 2 minutes Corpse Pose

STRAIGHT ARM FORWARD BEND p105 Hold 3 minutes

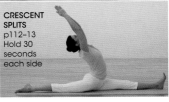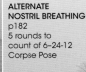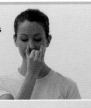

LATERAL BEND WITH TWIST p107 Hold 1 minute each side

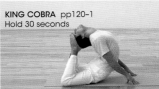

FULL SPINAL TWIST p149 Hold 30 seconds each side

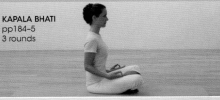

LOTUS PEACOCK p157 Hold 1 minute

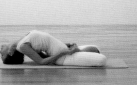

DANCING LORD SIVA pp160-1 Hold 1 minute each side

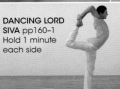

TRIANGLE: HEAD TO TOE p169 Hold 1 minute each side Final relaxation 8 minutes

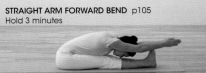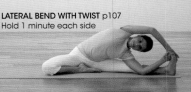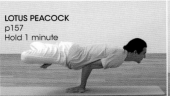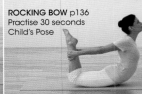

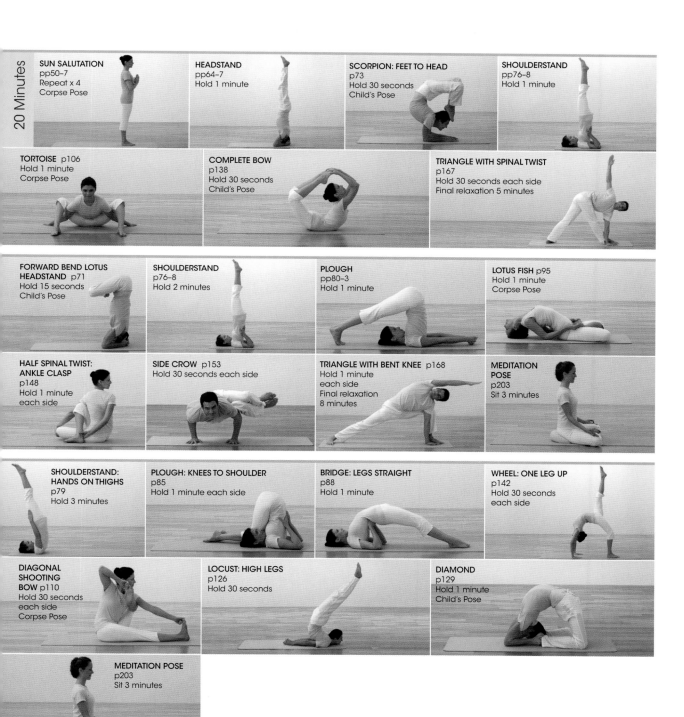

20 Minutes

SUN SALUTATION
pp50–7
Repeat x 4
Corpse Pose

HEADSTAND
pp64–7
Hold 1 minute

SCORPION: FEET TO HEAD
p73
Hold 30 seconds
Child's Pose

SHOULDERSTAND
pp76–8
Hold 1 minute

TORTOISE p106
Hold 1 minute
Corpse Pose

COMPLETE BOW
p138
Hold 30 seconds
Child's Pose

TRIANGLE WITH SPINAL TWIST
p167
Hold 30 seconds each side
Final relaxation 5 minutes

FORWARD BEND LOTUS HEADSTAND p71
Hold 15 seconds
Child's Pose

SHOULDERSTAND
p76–8
Hold 2 minutes

PLOUGH
pp80–3
Hold 1 minute

LOTUS FISH p95
Hold 1 minute
Corpse Pose

HALF SPINAL TWIST: ANKLE CLASP
p148
Hold 1 minute
each side

SIDE CROW p153
Hold 30 seconds each side

TRIANGLE WITH BENT KNEE p168
Hold 1 minute
each side
Final relaxation
8 minutes

MEDITATION POSE
p203
Sit 3 minutes

SHOULDERSTAND: HANDS ON THIGHS
p79
Hold 3 minutes

PLOUGH: KNEES TO SHOULDER
p85
Hold 1 minute each side

BRIDGE: LEGS STRAIGHT
p88
Hold 1 minute

WHEEL: ONE LEG UP
p142
Hold 30 seconds
each side

DIAGONAL SHOOTING BOW p110
Hold 30 seconds
each side
Corpse Pose

LOCUST: HIGH LEGS
p126
Hold 30 seconds

DIAMOND
p129
Hold 1 minute
Child's Pose

MEDITATION POSE
p203
Sit 3 minutes

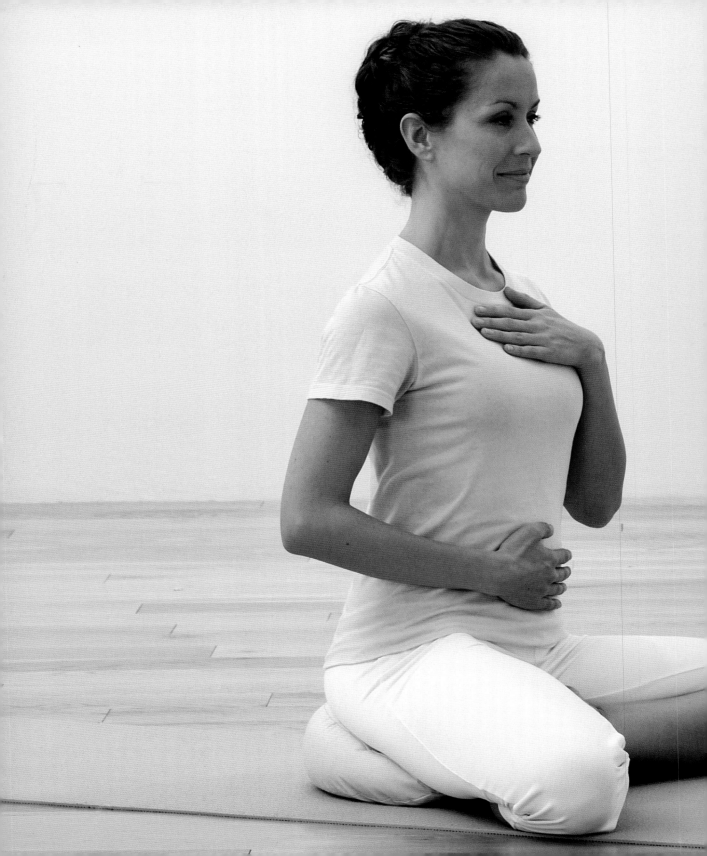

Proper Breathing

Pranayama

In the yogic tradition, the breath is seen as the outward manifestation of prana, or vital energy. Gaining control of the breath by practising breathing exercises – pranayama – increases the flow of prana through the body, which literally recharges body and mind. Aim to practise pranayama for up to 30 minutes daily, before or after asana practice.

Circulation of prana

According to the ancient yogic texts, prana circulates through the body in a network of 72,000 astral energy channels, or *nadis*. These not only permeate every part of the body, but also create an extensive energy field, or aura, around it. When you perform asanas, you apply pressure to points where important nadis cross. This works like acupressure, unblocking vital energy.

Strengthening the flow of prana

Yoga breathing exercises focus specifically on opening two major nadis – the *pingala* nadi and the *ida* nadi – and strengthening the flow of prana in them. The pingala nadi corresponds to the right nostril and left hemisphere of the brain, and the ida nadi to the left nostril and right brain. In the mystical language of yoga, the pingala nadi is warming and corresponds to *Ha*, or the sun; the ida is cooling and corresponds to *Tha*, or the moon. The final step of the eight-fold path of Hatha and Raja Yoga (see p11) comes about when there is perfect balance between these two nadis. The most important nadi, however, is the *sushumna*, which corresponds to the spinal cord. When the pingala and ida nadis are in balance, the sushumna opens, allowing vital energy to flow upwards and spiritual enlightenment to occur.

Training the respiratory muscles

Although the language and imagery of pranayama may appear quite mystical, in practice its effects are concrete. Whether you are a beginner or a more advanced yoga practitioner, pranayama trains the respiratory muscles, develops use of your lungs' full capacity, and improves your body's supply of oxygen while reducing its carbon dioxide levels. It also helps to relax and strengthen your nervous system, calm the mind, and improve concentration.

Begin your pranayama practice by lying in Corpse Pose (see p46) for 2–3 minutes. After your practice, relax in Corpse Pose again to release any tension in the hips or lower back from sitting cross-legged.

What is prana?

Prana, or vital energy, is found in all forms of life, from mineral to mankind, where its force controls and regulates every part of the body. Although prana is in all forms of matter, it is not matter. It is the energy that animates matter.

Prana is in the air, but it is not oxygen, nor any of its chemical constituents. It is in food, water, and sunlight, and yet it is not vitamin, heat, or light. Food, water, and air are only the media through which prana is carried. We absorb prana through the food we eat, the water we drink, and the air we breathe.

The easiest way to control prana is to regulate the breath – pranayama. Every part of the body can be filled with prana and when we do this, the entire body is under our control.

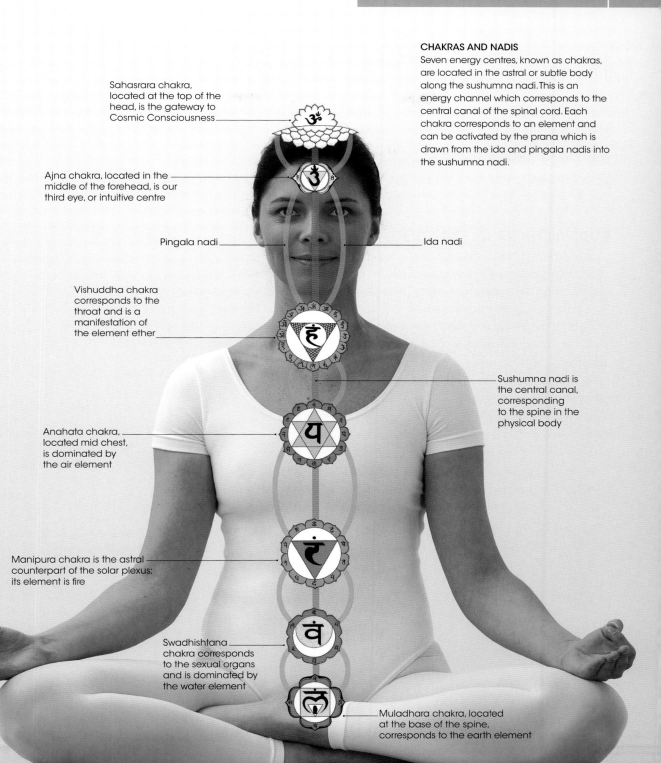

CHAKRAS AND NADIS
Seven energy centres, known as chakras, are located in the astral or subtle body along the sushumna nadi. This is an energy channel which corresponds to the central canal of the spinal cord. Each chakra corresponds to an element and can be activated by the prana which is drawn from the ida and pingala nadis into the sushumna nadi.

Sahasrara chakra, located at the top of the head, is the gateway to Cosmic Consciousness

Ajna chakra, located in the middle of the forehead, is our third eye, or intuitive centre

Pingala nadi

Ida nadi

Vishuddha chakra corresponds to the throat and is a manifestation of the element ether

Sushumna nadi is the central canal, corresponding to the spine in the physical body

Anahata chakra, located mid chest, is dominated by the air element

Manipura chakra is the astral counterpart of the solar plexus; its element is fire

Swadhishtana chakra corresponds to the sexual organs and is dominated by the water element

Muladhara chakra, located at the base of the spine, corresponds to the earth element

Preparatory exercises

Abdominal breathing is the essential preparatory technique to master before beginning any pranayama proper. This is the first stage on the road to the Full Yogic Breath, which teaches you how to make full use of your lungs' capacity. Once you can comfortably practise this, you are ready for the pranayama exercises on pp182–85.

Abdominal Breathing

Learning how to breathe deeply using your abdomen is one of the keys to pranayama. Practise it first when you relax in Corpse Pose (see p46) in preparation for your asana practice, and repeat it when you lie in Corpse Pose before your pranayama session. For several minutes, focus on slow, rhythmical breathing and the movement of your abdomen.

During Abdominal Breathing, the diaphragm draws air into and expels it from the lowest – and largest – part of the lungs. In order for the diaphragm to move freely, your abdominal muscles must be completely relaxed, so practise for a few minutes.

"If your body is strong and healthy with much prana, you will have a natural tendency to produce health and vitality in those close to you. "

Swami Vishnudevananda

Practising Abdominal Breathing

Lie in Corpse Pose (see p46), palms on your abdomen and fingers apart. As you breathe, feel the movement between your first rib, your navel, and your hips. Notice movement in the back of your body, too, around the kidneys and the lower back, and below your waist.

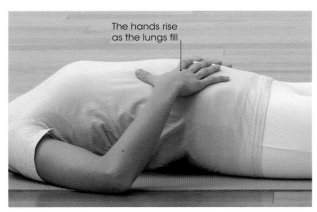
The hands rise as the lungs fill

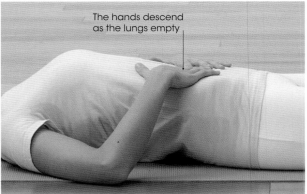
The hands descend as the lungs empty

INHALATION
Inhale for five seconds. As your abdomen expands, notice how your hands rise and your fingers draw apart.

EXHALATION
Exhale for five seconds. Notice your hands moving down and fingers coming together. Repeat the in- and out-breaths for two minutes.

Practising Full Yogic Breath

Positioning your hands on your abdomen and chest helps you learn to contract and relax the respiratory muscles in the correct order. If you find it easier, begin with a few breaths in Corpse Pose (see p46) before sitting up. Breathe very slowly throughout.

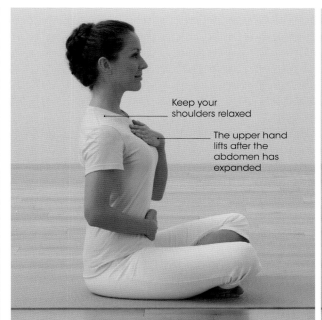

Keep your shoulders relaxed

The upper hand lifts after the abdomen has expanded

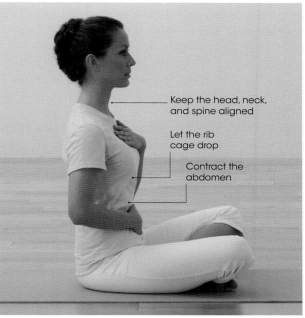

Keep the head, neck, and spine aligned

Let the rib cage drop

Contract the abdomen

INHALATION
Sit in a comfortable, cross-legged position and place one hand on your chest and the other on your abdomen. As you inhale, gradually expand the abdomen, then raise and open the rib cage, and finally lift the collar bones.

EXHALATION
Begin the exhalation by relaxing the abdomen, then lower the rib cage, and finally slightly contract the abdomen to actively empty the lungs. Repeat the inhalations and exhalations in this way for about two minutes.

Full Yogic Breath

This complete breath makes full use of your respiratory muscles. Learning to fill and empty the lungs to their maximum in a relaxed and controlled manner has a multitude of uses. It improves your muscle strength as you move into, hold, and release an asana. And when you perform a few cycles of the Full Yogic Breath during the short relaxation period between one asana and the next, it helps quickly to replenish the oxygen you have used while practising the asana. The muscle control you develop in the Full Yogic Breath – from the pelvis right up to the skull – also improves your awareness of spinal alignment in an asana. You might like to perform a few full yogic breaths as a quick pick-me-up at work, too, to help replenish your energy levels and quickly restore concentration.

Alternate Nostril Breathing

This is an excellent exercise for balancing the nervous system. Practising it can calm you down when you feel hyperactive, stimulate you when you feel lethargic, and centre you when you feel distracted. The prolonged exhalations release tension, the deep inhalations draw prana into the solar plexus and, when you retain the breath, prana is directed to the area of the third eye, bringing about mental poise.

How to practise

Pranayama should feel pleasant and never stressful. Beginners will find the ratio of inhalation to retention and exhalation in the complete technique too challenging, so start with Single Nostril Breathing before progressing through the levels. You will feel the benefits, no matter which level you practise at.

Single Nostril Breathing

Place your right hand in front of your face in Vishnu Mudra (see below, right). Close your right nostril with your thumb (see opposite). Inhale for three seconds and exhale for six seconds through your left nostril. This is one round. Practise up to ten rounds. Repeat on the other nostril: close your left nostril with your ring finger, and inhale and exhale through your right nostril. Practise ten rounds on each side regularly over a few weeks. Gradually increase the ratio of the exhalation to the inhalation – first inhale for four seconds and exhale for eight, then lengthen the ratio to 5:10, and finally to 6:12.

Simple Alternate Nostril Breathing

After mastering the 6:12 ratio of Single Nostril Breathing, move on to simple Alternate Nostril Breathing. Closing your right nostril with your thumb, inhale through your left nostril for four seconds, close your left nostril with your ring finger, open your right nostril and exhale through it for eight seconds. Inhale through your right nostril for four seconds, then exhale through your left nostril for eight seconds. Practise up to ten rounds. Gradually increase the inhalation:exhalation ratio to 5:10, then to 6:12, and finally to 7:14.

Alternate Nostril Breathing with Retention

Once you have mastered the 7:14 ratio of the simple Alternate Nostril Breathing, move on to Alternate Nostril Breathing with Breath Retention. Inhale through your left nostril for four seconds, close the nostril (see opposite), hold your breath for 8 seconds, then exhale through your right

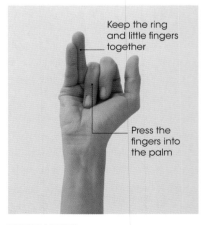

Keep the ring and little fingers together

Press the fingers into the palm

VISHNU MUDRA
Hold your right hand with the palm facing you and fold the first and second fingers into the palm. Try to keep your thumb and ring and little fingers straight.

Positioning the hand

Using a *mudra*, or energetic seal, like Vishnu Mudra (see opposite) helps to contain prana within the body, but is useful on a purely physical level, too, providing a tangible aid to concentration.

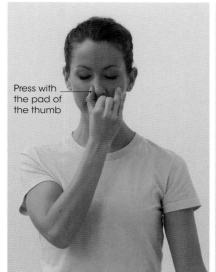

Press with the pad of the thumb

BREATHING THROUGH THE LEFT NOSTRIL
With your right hand in Vishnu Mudra (see opposite), close the right nostril with your thumb; inhale through the left nostril.

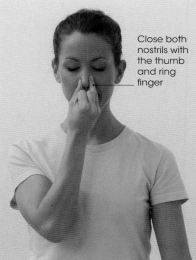

Close both nostrils with the thumb and ring finger

BREATH RETENTION
To retain your breath, close both nostrils with the thumb and the ring finger.

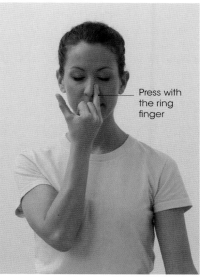

Press with the ring finger

BREATHING THROUGH THE RIGHT NOSTRIL
Close the left nostril with your ring finger, and exhale through the right nostril.

nostril for eight seconds. Then inhale through your right nostril for four seconds, hold your breath for eight seconds and exhale through your left nostril for eight seconds. Practise up to ten rounds. Increase the inhalation:retention:exhalation ratio to 5:10:10, then to 6:12:12, and finally to 7:14:14.

Complete Alternate Nostril Breathing

As you improve, try a longer breath retention – complete Alternate Nostril Breathing. Inhale through your left nostril for four seconds, hold the breath for sixteen seconds, and exhale through the right nostril for eight seconds. Then inhale through the right nostril for four seconds, hold the breath for eight seconds, and exhale through the left nostril for sixteen seconds. Practice up to ten rounds. Increase the inhalation:retention:exhalation ratio to 5:20:10, then to 6:24:12, and finally to 7:28:14.

Kapala Bhati

Literally translated as "shining skull", this exercise cleanses the respiratory passages, including the nasal passages in the head. It is one of the *kriyas*, or organ-cleansing exercises of Hatha and Raja Yoga (see pp10–11). Kapala Bhati also increases the capacity of the lungs, stimulates blood circulation, and gives a gentle massage to the heart. People who have asthma often find it helpful.

How to practise

Kapala Bhati consists of a series of short and active exhalations, alternated with passive, relaxed inhalations. The intense expulsions of stale air from the lungs increase the uptake of oxygen into the blood (see pp32–3), which can be felt especially in the brain. This makes Kapala Bhati an excellent way to improve your concentration, whether you are practising meditation or need a quick mental boost at work.

This exercise is best practised during a morning pranayama or meditation session; do not practise it late in the evening, since it activates the nervous system and may prevent you from falling asleep. If you are a beginner, do not try Kapala Bhati until you feel completely at ease practising Alternate Nostril Breathing with Breath Retention (see pp182–3).

Intermediate level

Sit with your legs crossed and your hands in Chin Mudra (see p204) and take a few slow, deep abdominal breaths. Notice the abdomen moving out as you inhale and in as you exhale. Then start a series of ten rhythmic, short, active exhalations (see opposite). After each active exhalation, let a gentle, passive in-breath just happen. The time taken for one exhalation and inhalation should be about two seconds.

After ten of these "pumps" out and in, take two slow full yogic breaths (see p181). Then inhale comfortably to 80 per cent of your capacity and hold the breath, according to your ability, for 20–60 seconds. Exhale slowly, with control. This is one round. After a few relaxed breaths, practise two more rounds.

Advanced level

Using the same technique, gradually increase the number of times you "pump" out and in per round to 50. You can speed up the rate at which you breathe, but never faster than one second for one exhalation and inhalation. As you become more relaxed and focused, try to hold the breath during the

Avoiding hyperventilation

When you practise Kapala Bhati for the first time, you may feel dizzy. This is caused by hyperventilation. If this happens, stop immediately, lie on your back and relax. Once the dizziness has gone, check whether you were making one of the following mistakes, and take the remedying action set out below.

The chest or collar bones move: Check that only your abdomen is moving during both exhalations and inhalations.

Your abdomen is not moving in when you exhale: Check that your abdomen is actively contracting and moving inwards every time you exhale.

You are inhaling too deeply or you are actively pushing out your abdomen: Inhale passively so that the abdomen simply moves forwards into its neutral position.

You are pumping too fast: You should reduce the speed of the pumping to 2 seconds for one inhalation and exhalation.

retention for up to 90 seconds. While you are holding your breath, focus on the third-eye area between your eyebrows. While you hold your breath, you may feel a pleasant warmth around your abdomen. This is the activated prana in your solar plexus. With each round of practice, the solar plexus recharges further, and prana starts moving up the spine. After sustained practice, you will find that the movement of prana is in accordance with how focused you are. The energy literally moves to where your thoughts go, which is why you should focus on the third eye.

Inhaling and exhaling

It is important to get the "pumping" technique right in this powerful exercise. Emphasize the exhalation; if you do this correctly, it creates a vacuum and the in-breath happens naturally, without requiring any effort.

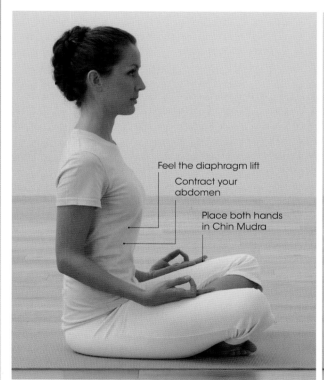

Feel the diaphragm lift

Contract your abdomen

Place both hands in Chin Mudra

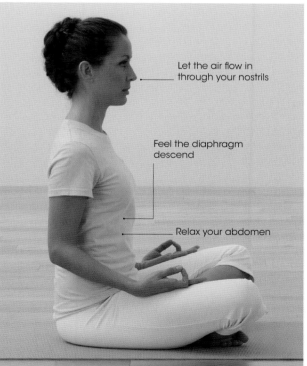

Let the air flow in through your nostrils

Feel the diaphragm descend

Relax your abdomen

ACTIVE EXHALATION
To actively exhale, firmly contract your abdomen and feel your diaphragm lift to push the air out of your lungs forcefully through both nostrils.

PASSIVE INHALATION
To exhale passively, simply release the abdomen. Feel the diaphragm descend and the air rush in. Do not try to take a breath; let the inhalation come easily, by itself.

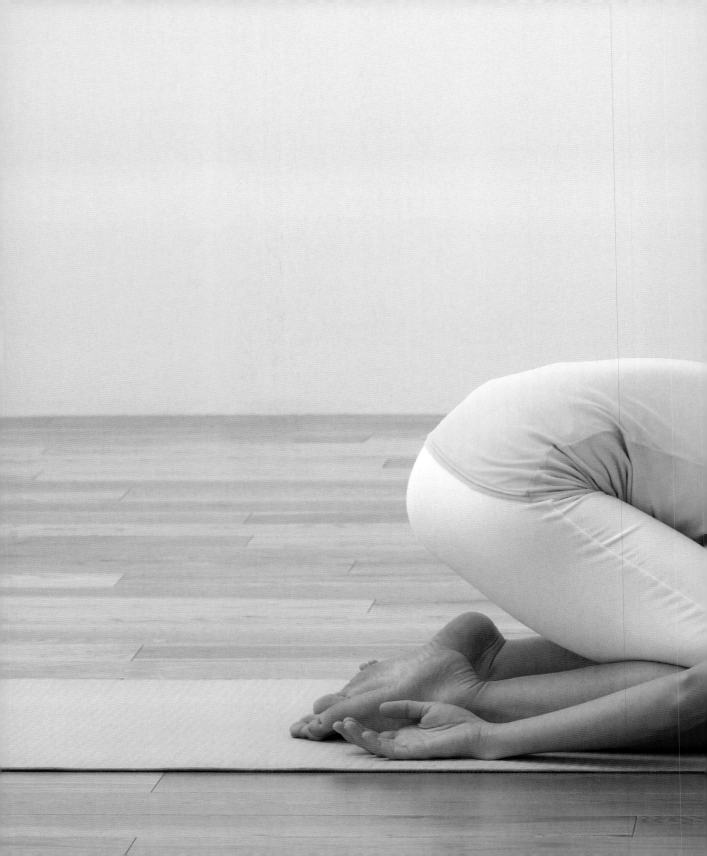

Proper Relaxation

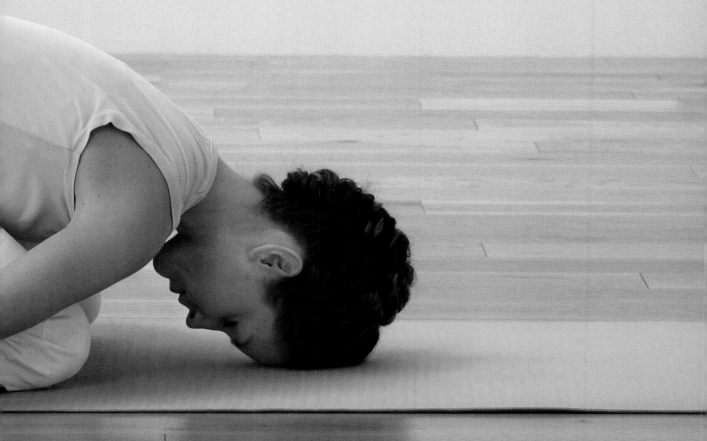

Relaxation between asanas

Take time to relax between one asana and the next – this allows the body to absorb the effects of the pose and be reinvigorated. Relax for a minimum of 8 deep breaths, but for no more than 2 minutes, so the body stays warm to progress to the next pose.

Why relax?

When you are performing postures, you can observe how the asana practice contains its own, in-built rhythmical alternation between effort and relaxation. In some asanas, your muscles are first stretched and then relaxed; in others, they are contracted and then relaxed (see p36). Relaxing between asanas confirms this pattern of effort and release in your nervous system, so that by the time you reach the final relaxation (see pp192–3), your nervous system is so well balanced that you will be able to relax simply by visualizing yourself relaxed – in other words, by using autosuggestion (see p194).

Relaxing on your back

Corpse Pose is the preferred position for relaxation between most asanas – exceptions are for backward bends and inversions. If you find this pose uncomfortable, use the alternative pose on the opposite page.

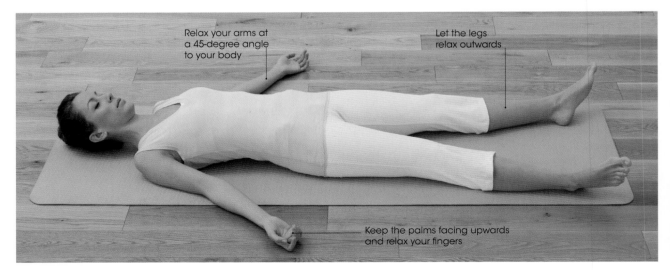

Relax your arms at a 45-degree angle to your body

Let the legs relax outwards

Keep the palms facing upwards and relax your fingers

CORPSE POSE
To get into Corpse Pose, follow the instructions for the initial relaxation (see p46). Take at least 8 deep, rhythmical breaths as you lie in Corpse Pose, and notice the effects of the pose you have just completed on your body and mind. Then progress to the next asana. If you find Corpse Pose uncomfortable, try the alternative positions opposite.

Alternative supine position

You may be uncomfortable lying on your back if you are unable to relax fully the muscles of the lower back. If this is the case, try the exercise below. After some practice, you will find that you can lie more comfortably in Corpse Pose to relax between asanas.

When Corpse Pose is uncomfortable

Bringing your knees towards your chest releases tension in the lower back. You can then drop your feet to the floor and practise the relaxation between asanas with your knees bent and your feet hip-width apart.

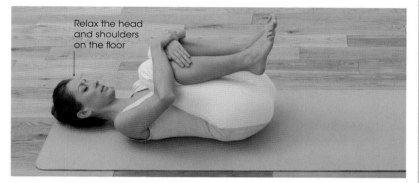

Relax the head and shoulders on the floor

HUGGING THE KNEES
1 Bend both legs and bring your knees towards your chest. Wrap your arms around your knees, and hold onto one wrist with the other hand. This gives the lower back a gentle stretch and releases tension around that part of the spine.

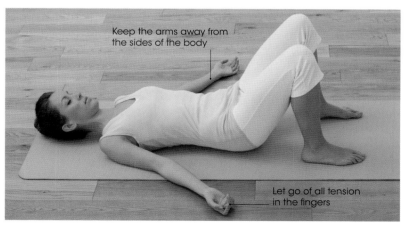

Keep the arms away from the sides of the body

Let go of all tension in the fingers

FEET ON FLOOR
2 Place your feet flat on the floor, about 20cm (8in) from your buttocks and relax your arms to the sides, with the palms facing upwards and the fingers completely relaxed. Take at least 8 deep, rhythmical breaths before progressing to the next asana.

"In order to regulate and balance the work of the body and mind, it is necessary to economize the energy produced by the body. This is the main purpose of learning how to relax."

Swami Vishnudevananda

Relaxing on your front

After asanas such as Cobra (see pp116–21) and Locust (see pp122–33), and variations performed from a prone position – lying on your abdomen – relax on your front before moving on to the next asana (see below). As you relax, notice the effect of the pose you have just performed on your body and mind, and feel the respiratory movement in your abdomen.

Relaxing on your abdomen

Turning your legs inwards in these prone relaxation positions creates rotation in the hip joints, which helps the muscles in the legs to relax. If your body feels tense or you get cramp in the feet in the basic position, try the alternative position (see below).

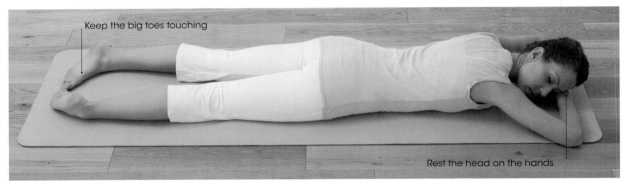

Keep the big toes touching

Rest the head on the hands

BASIC POSITION
Lie on your front with your arms folded in front of you and your hands one on top of the other. Turn your head to one side and rest it on your hands. This releases tension in the neck and shoulders and makes breathing more comfortable. The "pillow" formed by your hands takes any pressure away from your cheeks. Keep your legs slightly apart and turn your toes inwards. Take at least 8 deep, rhythmical breaths before progressing to the next asana.

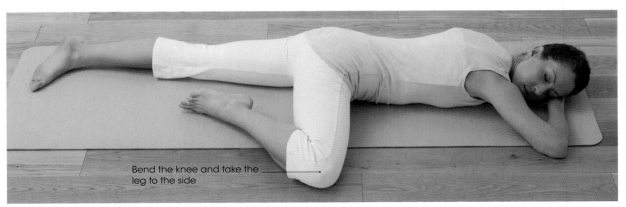

Bend the knee and take the leg to the side

ALTERNATIVE POSITION
Lie on your front with your arms folded in front of your head and your hands one on top of the other. Turn your head to one side and rest it on your hands. Keep your legs slightly apart and turn your toes inwards. Bend one knee and take the leg out to the side, towards your arm – this is Baby Krishna Pose. Keep your extended leg, your spine, and your head aligned. Take at least 8 deep, rhythmical breaths before progressing to the next asana.

Following Headstand (see pp62–75), Half Spinal Twist (see pp144–9), and any backward-bending asanas, relax in Child's Pose (see below). Child's Pose is good for relaxing the head and shoulders and gently stretching out the spine, which invigorates the nervous system. This pose also brings a refreshing flow of blood to the brain, for a rejuvenating effect before you move on to practise the next pose.

"We should not confuse relaxation with laziness. In infancy the child relaxes naturally; some adults possess this power of relaxation. Such persons are noted for their endurance, strength, vigour, and vitality."

Swami Vishnudevananda

Relaxing in a forward bend

The slight forward bend in Child's Pose gives your back and the muscles around your hips a soothing stretch. If you find it difficult to sit on your heels or your forehead does not reach the floor, practise the variation (see below).

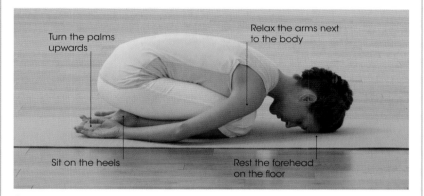

Turn the palms upwards

Relax the arms next to the body

Sit on the heels

Rest the forehead on the floor

CHILD'S POSE
Sit on your heels and lean forwards until your forehead comes to the floor. Extend your arms alongside your legs and rest your hands beside your feet, palms facing upwards. Take at least 8 deep, rhythmical breaths before progressing to the next asana.

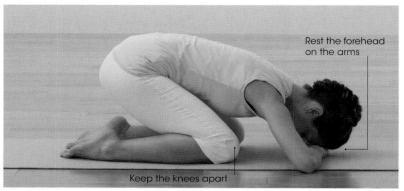

Rest the forehead on the arms

Keep the knees apart

CHILD'S POSE VARIATION
Sit on your heels with your knees slightly apart, lean forwards, and fold your arms on the floor in front of you, hands one on top of the other. Rest your forehead on your folded arms. Take at least 8 deep, rhythmical breaths before progressing to the next asana.

Final Relaxation

At the end of every yoga session, you should practise a final relaxation lasting 15–20 minutes. This will bring about complete physical, mental, and spiritual relaxation, which is a key experience of yoga.

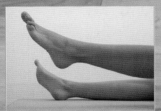

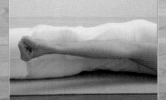

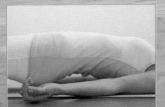

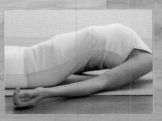

1 Inhale and lift your right leg 10cm (4in) off the mat. Hold your breath for a few seconds, tense your leg, then exhale and allow your leg to drop. Repeat with the left leg.

2 Inhale and lift both arms 10cm (4in) off the mat. Hold your breath for a few seconds, tense your arms, then exhale and allow your arms to drop to the mat.

3 Inhale and lift your hips and buttocks off the mat. Hold your breath for a few seconds, tense your buttocks, then exhale and release.

4 Inhale and lift your chest off the mat. Hold your breath for a few seconds, tense your shoulder blades, then exhale and release.

Allow the feet to fall outwards

Following the sequence

Your blood pressure and body temperature will drop during final relaxation so, depending on the season, you may like to cover yourself loosely with a blanket before you begin. Follow Steps 1–8 below to achieve a comfortable Corpse Pose, then use the physical, mental, and spiritual relaxation exercises on pages 194–5 in the suggested order. Then slowly stretch and sit for a minute cross-legged to end your practice with the mantra "OM".

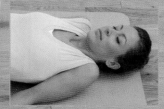

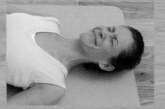

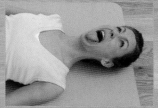

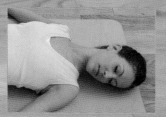

5 Inhale and pull your shoulders towards your ears. Hold your breath for a few seconds, then exhale and release your shoulders.

6 Inhale and squeeze the muscles of your face tightly together. Hold your breath for a few seconds, then exhale and release.

7 Inhale, open your mouth, stick your tongue out, and look to your forehead. Hold your breath for a few seconds, then exhale and release.

8 With an inhalation, slowly roll your head to one side; with an exhalation, roll it to the other side. End by bringing your head back to centre.

Breathe very slowly and gently in the abdomen

Let go of any tension in the face

Let the weight of the head sink into the mat

Relax the shoulders into the mat

Relax the palms and fingers

Complete yogic relaxation

Yogic relaxation has three aspects: physical relaxation, mental relaxation, and spiritual relaxation. As you lie in Corpse Pose for your final relaxation (see pp192–3), practise the thought-focusing exercises below to relax body, mind, and spirit.

Part 1: Physical relaxation

Take a few slow, rhythmic breaths using your abdomen (see p180). Then follow this exercise in autosuggestion for five to ten minutes. Have a clear mental picture of your feet, think about the downward pull of gravity, then send a mental command to your feet by silently saying, "I am relaxing my feet, I am relaxing my feet, my feet are relaxed." Move up the body; each time clearly visualize the area you are focusing on, think about the pull of gravity and your rhythmic breathing, then send a command to relax to your ankles, calves, knees and thighs, hips and buttocks, abdomen and chest, lower back, middle back, shoulders and neck, hands and fingers, arms, mouth and

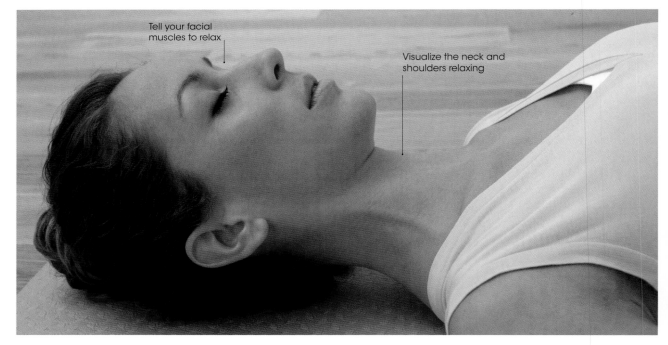

Tell your facial
muscles to relax

Visualize the neck and
shoulders relaxing

PHYSICAL RELAXATION
Each time you move on consciously to relax another part of the body, make sure you have a clear mental picture of that area before tuning your thoughts into the downward pull of gravity and the rhythmical flow of your breath. Finally, give the mental command to relax by silently repeating the phrase beginning "I am relaxing...".

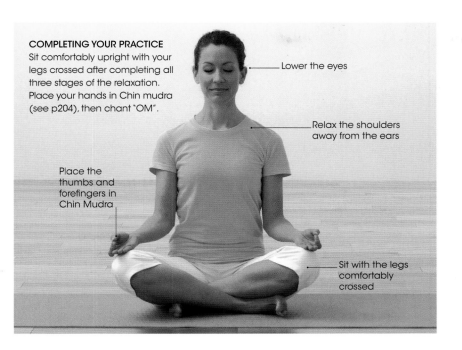

COMPLETING YOUR PRACTICE
Sit comfortably upright with your legs crossed after completing all three stages of the relaxation. Place your hands in Chin mudra (see p204), then chant "OM".

Lower the eyes

Relax the shoulders away from the ears

Place the thumbs and forefingers in Chin Mudra

Sit with the legs comfortably crossed

"During spiritual relaxation the Yogi identifies himself with the all-pervading, all-powerful, all-peaceful and joyful self within himself, the real source of knowledge and strength"

Swami Vishnudevananda

eyes, facial muscles and scalp. Finally, relax your internal organs. Again, visualize the area, breathe slowly, and send the command to relax to one organ at a time: kidneys, liver, intestines, bladder, pancreas, stomach, heart, lungs, and brain. Your subconscious mind conveys the command.

Part 2: Mental relaxation

The mind is always moving between the past and the future, and in the present it is constantly pulled by the five senses. It needs to relax, so practise this mental relaxation for about two minutes. Continue abdominal breathing, this time inhaling and exhaling for five seconds each. The speed and rhythm of your breath and your thought waves are intimately linked. Start to observe the flow of air moving in and out of your nostrils. Soon your mind will be calm; if you sense it becoming active, focus on your breathing until it quietens.

Part 3: Spiritual relaxation

Complete spiritual relaxation is possible only if your thoughts have a carefree focus, so now visualize a calm lake, unruffled by waves. Picture the still water resting on your inner self, which is timeless and unchanging. Continue for five to eight minutes. Then take a few deep breaths, slowly move your legs and arms, and give your whole body a good stretch. Finally, spend a minute sitting cross-legged and chant the mantra "OM". Now you will be able to hold this sense of relaxation and focus for several hours.

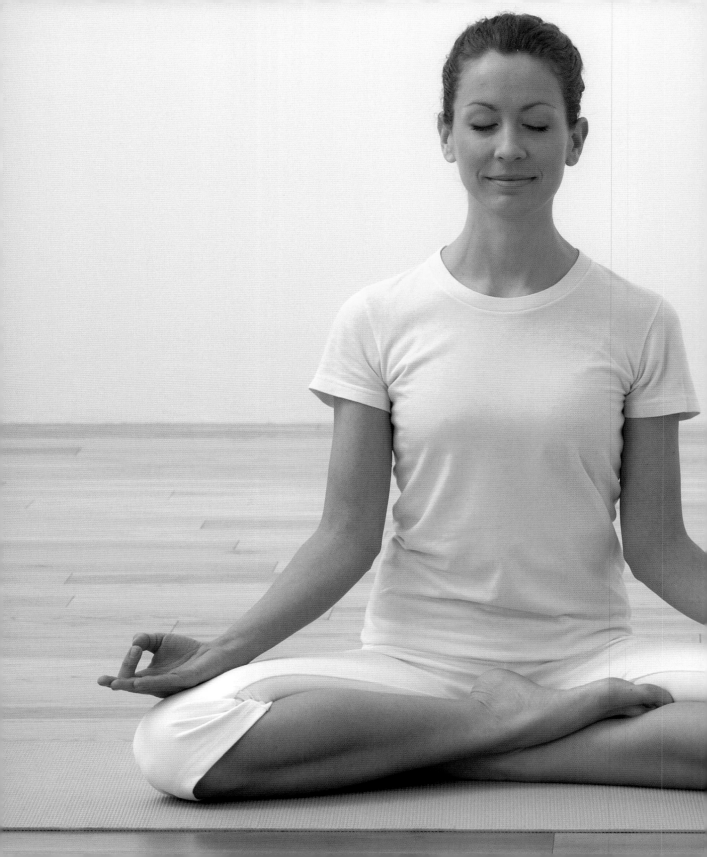

Positive Thinking and Meditation

Why meditate?

Meditation lies at the heart of any yoga practice. Once you feel comfortable practising the asanas and breathing exercises, you will feel more relaxed in your body. Then, it will seem like a natural step to pay more attention to your mind by practising meditation. This brings about greater mental and emotional balance and, eventually, inner peace.

Physical benefits

During meditation, the distractions of the world around you disappear and the parasympathetic nervous system (see pp34–5) gently brings about a sense of relaxation and balance. Your heartbeat and respiratory rate slow and your internal organs are rested. Research shows that meditation stimulates the immune system, too, promoting health and protecting against illness.

Adepts of yoga have long recognized that the vibrations generated by thoughts and emotions affect every cell in the body – and that negative thoughts can impede the cells' capacity for regeneration and homeostasis (see p206). The focus in meditation on positive and harmonious thoughts, therefore, is thought to promote health and well-being at a cellular level.

Mental benefits

Ancient yogis aptly compared an unfocused mind to a crazy, drunken monkey, jumping from one thought to the next in a never-ending cycle. It's all but impossible to stop the mind leaping from one thought to another. During meditation, you simply learn how to focus on the present. This prevents your mind from dwelling on the past or worrying about the future.

As your mind becomes more focused, confusion gives way to clarity. You find that you can face the conflicts that disturb your mental peace and you discover creative, positive solutions to those conflicts. This brings about a greater feeling of self-control, inner satisfaction, and sense of purpose.

What is more, you not only experience these benefits during meditation practice. They spill over into the rest of the day, helping you to concentrate better at work and play. By encouraging emotional balance and more patience and understanding, meditation also improves your relations with those around you. You will become less irritated by other people's habits, more understanding, and better able to accept their limitations.

The ultimate goal of meditation

Ancient yogic scriptures describe the goal of meditation as *samadhi*, or cosmic consciousness.

In this state of calm understanding, the illusion of ego (the feeling that you are separate from the world) vanishes. Everything dissolves into one consciousness, or Supreme Self. In this state, you might think, "I am not my body or my mind. My mind is only my story, and I am not my story. My body does not separate me from others. I am never alone, but always one with all." All negative emotions and limiting ideas about your body and inner self vanish, setting you free from discontent. You become aware of the purpose of life and, ultimately, lose fear of death.

Experienced yogis aim to be in this state at all times, living life as one unbroken meditation. As a beginner, start by shaking free the deep-rooted habit of identifying with everything in your mind. This takes practice, but as the saying goes, every journey of a thousand miles starts with a single step.

Spiritual benefits

As your meditation practice deepens, you will gain glimpses of a state of being that you have probably never experienced before. You may feel as if life's clouds have dissipated and you can see more blue sky. You will have a sense of greater inner space, well-being, positivity, and a real feeling of trust in the goodness of life. You will start to realize that beyond the familiar world of thoughts and emotions lies a whole new realm of consciousness. Your sense of yourself will expand beyond an awareness of your body and your mind and, ultimately, you will experience a feeling of unity with everything around you.

Meditation is so powerful that its benefits extend far beyond the person who is meditating. Yogis believe that the powerful vibrations of peace that emanate from an experienced meditator have a positive effect on everyone that person comes into contact with – and that, in the end, they influence the whole world. And so making your mind peaceful through meditation is the most positive thing you can do to contribute to world peace.

"Meditation is 'the cessation of mental activities'. When your thoughts reduce by just 20 per cent, you will experience relief and a sense of self-control."
Swami Sivananda

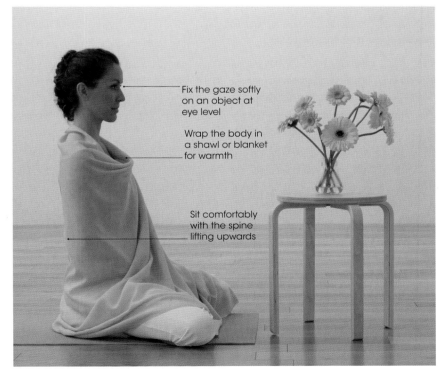

Fix the gaze softly on an object at eye level

Wrap the body in a shawl or blanket for warmth

Sit comfortably with the spine lifting upwards

SITTING TO MEDITATE
When you sit to practise meditation, your physical body is the first to relax. Once you feel settled, the mind begins to slow down, bringing the object of your concentration into sharper focus.

The art of concentration

Before you can learn to meditate, you have to be able to concentrate the mind. We can all concentrate to some degree, but the way we live and work today – constantly on call thanks to mobile technology and immersed in a sound-bite culture – means that many of us have only a short attention span. Practising the simple exercises on these pages will help to lengthen your attention span and enhance your ability to concentrate, which can boost the memory and benefit your psychological health.

What is concentration?

Concentration means attending fully to one thought or object for a substantial length of time. You are concentrating when you become engrossed in a book, eat without thinking about work, or forget about your home life when in the office. The ability to concentrate is not only essential for meditation, it is key to success in any endeavour, and once you have trained yourself to concentrate effectively, you can use the skill in many other areas of life. For example, being able to shut out other thoughts and not make haphazard or hasty decisions will make you more effective at work.

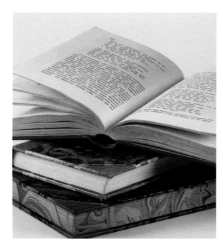

LOSE YOURSELF IN A BOOK
Read two or three pages of a book, giving them your full attention. Then test your concentration by stopping at the end of a page. How much do you remember of the story? Can you classify, group, or compare the facts you have been reading about?

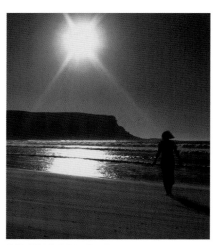

CONTEMPLATE NATURE
During the day, concentrate on the sky. Feel your mind expand as you reflect on its vast expanse. At night, concentrate on the moon or stars. By the sea, focus on waves. Or shift your gaze between objects near and far, such as a nearby tree and distant mountain.

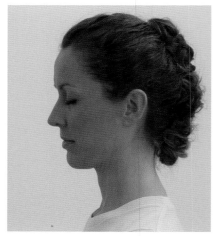

LISTEN TO A SOUND
Listen carefully to the ticking of a watch. When your mind wanders, bring it back to the sound. How long can you concentrate on that sound? Or listen to a prominent sound for a while, without reacting to it. Then shift your attention to other sounds, one by one.

The benefits of concentration

Practising concentration has many benefits. It can strengthen "thought-currents" – how we connect thoughts and ideas in the brain – making it easier to grasp difficult, complex, or confusing concepts. It also clarifies ideas, so you can express yourself more clearly. Concentration exercises energize the mind, boosting efficiency at work and in other tasks, while building will-power and the ability to influence other people positively. They also bring about serenity, insight, and cheerfulness.

Practical exercises

The exercises below provide an easy way to start developing your ability to concentrate. Initially, train your mind to concentrate on external objects, such as a book, sound, or something in nature, from waves on the ocean to stars in the sky. As you progress, you will be able to concentrate on more subtle subjects, such as an inner sound or an abstract idea. While practising, notice how aware you are of the various qualities of the experience when the mind is focused. Then note how difficult it is to assimilate an experience with an unfocused mind. When your mind wanders – which it will do often – remind it to come back to contemplation of the object or quality you are focusing on. Gradually lengthen your practice until you can concentrate for half an hour.

"Emotional balance maintained in all activities is the true sign of progress..."
Swami Sivananda

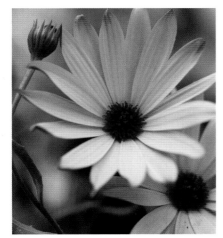

FOCUS ON A FLOWER
Sit comfortably with your eyes closed. Imagine a garden with many flowers. Gradually, bring your attention to a single flower. Visualize its colour and explore its other qualities, such as texture, shape, and scent. Concentrate on the flower's qualities for as long as possible.

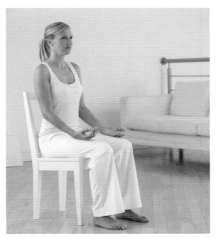

REFLECT ON AN IDEA
Relax your body and mind and think about a quality, such as compassion. Imagine how you could express it in your life. Think of great people who embodied it. Ask the quality to fill your heart, then to flow out to the whole world. Think of yourself as perfectly compassionate.

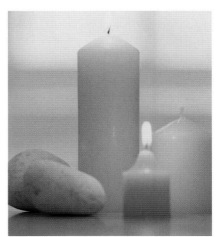

CANDLE CONTEMPLATION
Sit cross-legged in a dark room with a lighted candle at eye-level, an arm's distance away. Watch your breath for 2–3 minutes. Then look at the flame for 1 minute. Try not to blink. Close your eyes and visualize the flame between your eyebrows for a minute.

Practising meditation

Meditation is a state of relaxed awareness. Swami Vishnudevananda used to say that it is not possible to teach someone how to achieve this state, any more than it is possible to teach someone how to sleep. However, the more care and attention you give to your preparation for meditation, the more positive the results will be. This preparation can be divided into two parts: first become comfortable with physical meditation, then focus your mind with mental meditation (see p204).

Physical meditation

If you get the atmosphere right for meditation, the purity of the space will be so tangible that at times of stress you can sit in your meditation space, practise for half an hour, and experience great comfort and relief.

PLACE It's best to set aside a special room for meditation, but if this is not possible, try to separate one portion of a room to use for your practice. Keep it clean and tidy, and make a focal point by placing a candle and a spiritually uplifting picture at eye level in front of the place you sit for meditation. Gazing at the steady candle flame before starting a meditation practice helps to concentrate your mind and turn it inwards. Burning incense can also help to create a meditative mood. You will need a clean mat or folded woollen blanket to sit on. Many yogis like to place it to face North or East to take advantage of favourable magnetic vibrations. With repeated practice, the vibrations created during meditation will build a magnetic aura. Within six months, the peace and purity of the atmosphere should be tangible.

TIME The best times for meditation are at dawn and dusk, when the atmosphere is thought to be charged with a special spiritual force. At dawn, in the quiet hours after sleep, the mind is especially clear and unruffled. If this hour is tricky, practise at dusk or just before going to bed. Alternatively, find a time when you are free from daily activities and your mind can be calm.

HABIT Practise every day at the same time. As your subconscious mind gets accustomed to the regularity, you will find it easier to settle and focus. Start with 15 to 20 minutes, building up to one hour (aim for at least 30 minutes). It is better to meditate every day for 30 minutes than once a week for two hours.

"Feel the silence, hear the silence, touch and taste the silence. Silence is the music of your soul."

Swami Vishnudevananda

SITTING POSITION Sit on the floor to meditate, in a position that you can maintain comfortably, keeping your spine and neck straight but not tense. You do not have to sit in the classic Lotus posture – a simple, cross-legged pose makes a firm base, or you can sit in Half-lotus pose (see below). Sitting on a cushion helps the thighs to relax and brings the knees closer to the ground. In all these sitting positions, the legs make a triangular pattern. This shape contains the energy raised during meditation rather than allowing it to disperse in all directions.

If you can't sit on the floor easily, sit on a comfortable chair with your ankles crossed. Do not lie down to meditate – you will relax too completely and may fall asleep. Choose one of the three hand positions shown on p204.

BREATHING Once you are sitting comfortably, relax your body as much as possible, especially the muscles of the face, neck, and shoulders. Broaden your chest and lift your rib cage to encourage Abdominal Breathing (see p180), which brings oxygen to the brain. Then inhale and exhale rhythmically for about 3 seconds each, slowing your breath to an imperceptible rate. Notice how your breath becomes lighter and completely silent.

Sitting positions

Whichever position you choose, make sure it is comfortable – you should be able to sit with a straight spine without fidgeting for up to 30 minutes. If you find these poses too stressful on your hips or knees, sit on a chair. Then choose a hand position (see p204).

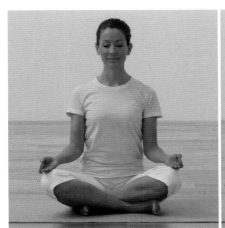

CROSS-LEGGED POSE
Sit comfortably upright and bend your knees, crossing one shin in front of the other. Try to relax your knees towards the floor.

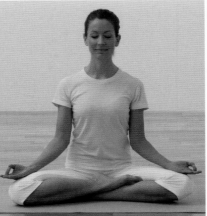

HALF-LOTUS POSE
Sit comfortably with your legs wide and bend one knee, bringing the sole against your groin. Place the opposite foot on top of the bent leg.

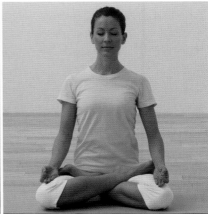

LOTUS POSE
Sit with crossed legs. Raise your front leg and place the top of the foot on the opposite thigh. Carefully lift the other foot onto the other thigh.

Hand positions

Once you are sitting comfortably, lift your spine and relax your shoulders. Rest your hands in one of these hand gestures, or *mudras*, to keep the arms and shoulders relaxed and to focus your prana, or vital energy.

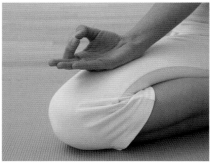

CHIN MUDRA
Rest the backs of your palms on your knees or thighs and join the tips of your thumbs and forefingers. Extend the other fingers.

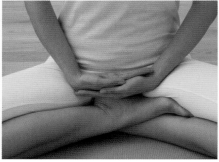

CUPPED HANDS
Turn both palms to face upwards in front of your groin and gently cup the back of your right hand in your left palm.

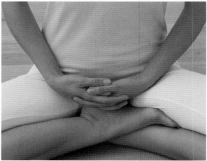

CLASPED HANDS
Turn both palms to face upwards in front of your groin and interlink your fingers, resting one thumb on top of the other,

Mental meditation

Follow these meditation techniques to stabilize your mental energy and to focus your mind. But first, simply allow your mind to wander. If, initially, you are too eager to control your mind, you might develop a headache.

GIVE THE MIND SPACE Focus deeply on your breathing to give your mind space. Then watch your mind closely. Be patient and compassionate with it: developing a trusting relationship with your mind ensures its co-operation.

DISASSOCIATE If your mind wanders, watch it objectively, as if watching a film. Just observe your thoughts for a few minutes and they will diminish.

CONCENTRATION POINT Bring your awareness to a *chakra* (see p179). If you relate easily to others, focus on the heart centre (*anahata* chakra), at the centre of your chest. If you are analytical, focus on the self-awareness centre (*ajna* chakra), between your eyebrows. Aim to keep this focus for life.

CONCENTRATION OBJECT Focus on a symbol; try something concrete, such as the sun or sky, or a positive quality, like love or compassion. Or try a mantra, such as "OM". Repeat the sound mentally, in time with your breath.

"During meditation, we watch our mind without expectation. Sustained attention combined with detachment ultimately unveils the ocean of wisdom that lies within"

Swami Vishnudevananda

Managing stress

It is now widely acknowledged, even by mainstream medicine, that meditation is very useful for treating depression and stress-related conditions. To understand how this works, it is helpful to know about the physiological changes that occur when we are feeling stressed, known as the "fight or flight response". This programming helped ancient man to deal with emergencies requiring a huge amount of physical effort, such as fighting off an animal.

The body's stress response

The "fight or flight response" activates the nervous system, and chemicals are released into the bloodstream, among them adrenaline, noradrenaline, and cortisol. These increase your rate of breathing, dilate your pupils to sharpen your eyesight, and direct blood away from your digestive system towards your muscles, readying the body for physical effort. Thanks to these changes, your reflexes quicken, you feel less pain, and your immune system gets ready for action. You suddenly perceive everything as a threat to survival, and are quick to react with anger or aggression and less likely to behave positively. We once needed such responses to ward off physical danger, but today, most stress is psychological, caused by work or relationships. And where in the past stress was resolved by fighting or running away, it now may not have a clear end. If the nervous system does not get a message that danger has passed, the "fight or flight response" persists; over time, this causes burnout.

COMBATING STRESS For your body to function well again, you must activate the parasympathetic nervous system (see p34–7). You can do this by following the physical preparation for meditation (see pp202–203), sitting quietly and breathing rhythmically. Then use the mental preparation techniques (see opposite) to relax your mind, focus it on a positive goal, and distance it from the stressor. You might also like to use positive affirmations to view your situation in a new light. Try saying, "I allow myself to relax. I am alive and I can breathe. This situation is temporary and will end. Help is available." Then focus your mind on a peaceful natural scene, a harmonious sound, or a pleasant memory. Or visualize a sage or saint, and feel powerful, soothing vibrations entering your heart. This creates a calm sense of connection with something greater than yourself, giving you confidence to deal with the causes of stress.

Stress-busting tools

Start dealing with symptoms of stress as soon as you notice them using these simple strategies.

Counter shallow breathing by taking a few deep abdominal breaths (see p180). Use your diaphragm fully and make the exhalations long.

Sit comfortably on a chair with your back straight, feet on the floor, palms on your thighs, and your eyes closed. Breathe deeply, and bring your attention to areas of your body in which you feel tension. Ask each part to relax. Repeat three times with full attention and confidence.

If you work long hours at a computer, practise eye exercises (see p48) two to three times a day and regularly look at the sky through a window.

If you sit for most of the day, get up every hour and do some stretches. Bend forwards for a few seconds, then bend backwards. Twist to the right, then to the left. Finally, stretch sideways.

Ease out any stress in the neck by practising neck rolls (see p49).

The law of karma

In yoga, the purpose of meditation is linked to the law of karma – the belief that everything happens for a reason and that every action has a reaction. Your meditation practice will guide your mind towards the positive thinking that will attract joy into your life. Swami Sivananda advised people to focus on a single positive quality for a whole month – the chart opposite will help you to do just that.

What is karma?

The law of action and reaction teaches that doing good deeds attracts goodness to us and, conversely, that doing bad deeds attracts ill. This is true of thoughts as well as deeds. The reaction provoked by a thought will be of the same nature and quality as the thought itself, so a negative thought attracts a negative reaction and a positive thought a positive one. Today, we tend to believe that others are responsible for what happens to us, especially for the more challenging episodes. We are quick to blame parents, teachers, or society at large for our ills. We fail to realize that our negative thoughts and emotions – fear of failure, resentment, anger, self-hatred – generate powerful, negative vibrations. These attract negative energy that influences events, the people we meet, and even the diseases we get. For example, dwelling on unhappy memories and worrying that painful things will happen again sets up a vibration of fear, which attracts fear and pain. This is the law of karma.

BEING RESPONSIBILE FOR YOUR LIFE Understanding the law of karma brings the realization that you are responsible for your own life. It is no use blaming others or outside events for the ills you suffer. The secret of happiness and pain rests in your hands – or, rather, in your mind. If the universe brings you only and exactly those things that are on the same wavelength as your thoughts and feelings, the key to happiness is to pay attention to what you think and feel. You are the architect of your own destiny. So if you find yourself thinking a negative thought, try to correct it quickly with a more positive one.

A HABIT OF POSITIVE THINKING Whenever possible, think joyous, happy, and harmonious thoughts. Yogis believe that these bring well-being to mind and body. Practising meditation is a good way to guide your mind towards the positive; if you practise in the early morning, the effects remain with you all day. Or you could repeat the positive affirmation of the day (see opposite).

"Yogis insist that the mind can and should be very dynamic and that it is the quality of our inner world that determines the quality of our lives."
Swami Sivadasananda

A year of positive thinking

Start each day by concentrating on the quality of the month, shown below. Allow its energy to vibrate in your mind and visualize the benefits of interacting with others using this quality. Repeat once during the day, then end your day with a short meditation on that thought. By the end of a month, you will have developed a habit of positive thinking.

JANUARY	FEBRUARY	MARCH	APRIL
Patience "I trust that life will bring me what I need."	Compassion "I have compassion for all beings."	Adaptability "I adapt easily to new circumstances."	Cheerfulness "I meet each situation with a cheerful mind."

MAY	JUNE	JULY	AUGUST
Love "I intend to greet each person with love."	Peace "My mind remains peaceful in all circumstances."	Courage "I am full of courage."	Will "My will is all-powerful."

SEPTEMBER	OCTOBER	NOVEMBER	DECEMBER
Humility "I surrender to the cosmic will."	Detachment "I look at my life circumstances from a new perspective."	Self-confidence "I trust that my inner self is pure positivity."	Endurance "I regard all difficulties as opportunities to grow."

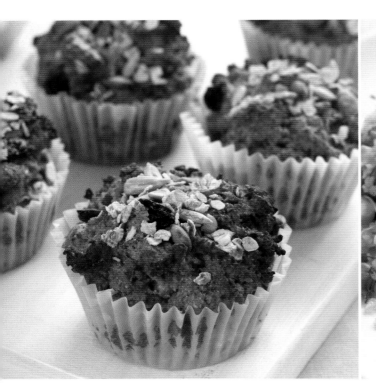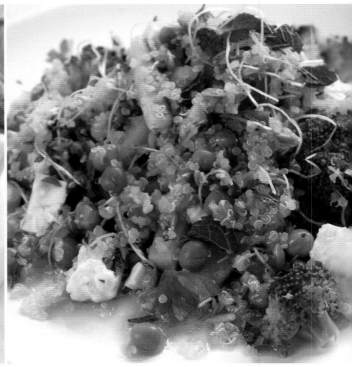

Proper Diet

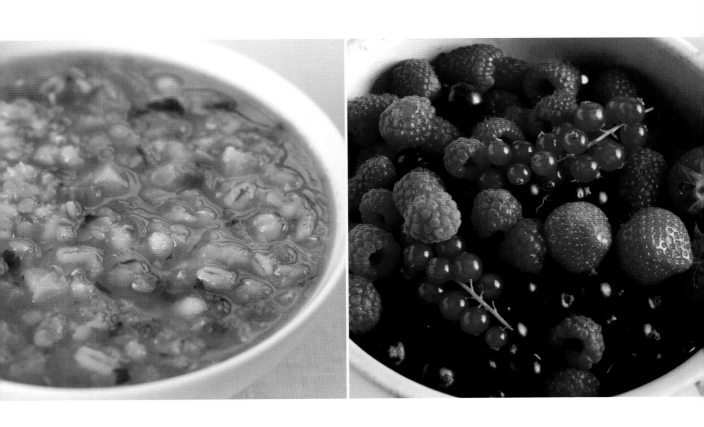

Yoga and Vegetarianism

The yogic tradition advocates a lacto-vegetarian diet – avoiding meat, fish, and eggs, and limiting your dairy intake. Predominantly plant-based, this diet ensures that your food gets its energy direct from the sun, the source of all life. Your food should also be freshly prepared and, ideally, organic.

Why be a vegetarian?

According to yogic tradition, a non-vegetarian diet violates the principle of ahimsa, the sanctity of all living things. But there are also many health benefits to vegetarianism. Research shows that vegetarians living in affluent countries enjoy remarkably good health and live longer than their meat-eating counterparts. They are slimmer, have lower blood pressure, and suffer less from heart disease, diabetes, dementia, and many cancers.

THE PROBLEM WITH MEAT Meat contains large amounts of cholesterol, saturated fat, and potentially carcinogenic (cancer-forming) compounds, including pesticide residues. When meat is grilled or fried, it forms carcinogenic polycyclic aromatic hydrocarbons, while cured and smoked meats contain nitrates and nitrites that may increase the risk of cancer, particularly among children. The findings of the China Study in 2006 indicated that the lower the percentage of animal-based foods in the diet, the greater the health benefits, and that getting one's nutrients from plant-based foods reduces the development of cancerous tumours.

Another concern about meat is that crowded factory farms are fertile breeding grounds for salmonella, e.coli, listeria, and campylobacter. What is more, the hormones, antibiotics, and vaccines that are given to animals leave residues that are believed to pose a threat to human health.

THE BENEFITS OF PLANT FOODS Plant foods contain dramatically higher amounts of antioxidants, fibre, and vitamins. They also contain phytonutrients that appear to offer protection against many cancers, assist in hormone balance, protect the heart, and help reduce blood pressure.

Following a vegetarian diet also offers a way of living an environmentally conscious lifestyle. Just think of this: it takes 11,000 litres (2500 gallons) of water to produce 500g (1lb) of meat, but only 110 litres (25 gallons) to produce 500g (1lb) wheat. It's easy to see why many argue that the most efficient way to feed the world's population is with a vegetarian diet.

Getting Your Calcium

Calcium is essential for bone health and to ensure efficient muscle contraction and blood clotting. If you are following a lacto-vegetarian diet, you have a number of options for getting enough calcium in your diet.

Everyone needs to eat 6–8 servings daily of foods that are rich in calcium. Below are foods that will give you 1 serving of a calcium-rich food:
- 120g (4¼oz) cooked quinoa
- 115g (4oz) cooked or 230g (8oz) raw broccoli, kale, bok choy, okra, or spinach
- 30ml (1fl oz) tahini
- 100g (3½oz) tofu
- 125ml (4fl oz) cow's milk, yogurt, or fortified soya milk
- 130g (6oz) dried apricots or currants

THE LACTO-VEGETARIAN FOOD PYRAMID

This vegetarian food pyramid is based on the latest research and reflects the total daily nutritional needs of an average adult woman. If you lead an active lifestyle, exercising regularly 2–3 times a week, you will need to increase your intake of all food groups. If you are older or less active, you will need to decrease your intake.

The foundation of the pyramid is wholegrains – the mainstay of a healthy vegetarian diet. The average adult woman should eat 6 servings daily. Next come pulses, dairy, nuts, and seeds – aim for 5 servings daily. The next largest intake is vegetables – aim for 4 servings daily. These are the most important source of vitamins, minerals, and phytonutrients. Next comes fruit – aim for 2 servings daily. Finally, eat fats and oils sparingly – not more than 2 servings daily.

Fats and oils

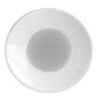

OLIVE OIL
2 servings, any
vegetable oil = 10ml
(½fl oz/2 tsp)

AN EASY MEASURE FOR SERVINGS

The cup measurements refer to American cups, which are an easy way to measure ingredients. You can also use a standard measuring jug in the same way, as follows:
1 cup = 230ml (8 fl oz)
½ cup = 115ml (4 fl oz)
¼ cup = 55ml (2 fl oz)

Fruit

 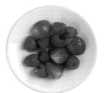

APPLES
1 serving, raw =
90g (3oz)

BERRIES
1 serving, any soft fruit
= 75g (3oz/½ cup)

Vegetables

RED PEPPERS
1 serving, raw =
90g (3oz/1 cup)

BROCCOLI
1 serving, raw =
90g (3oz/1 cup)

SALAD LEAVES
1 serving, any green
salad = 35g
(1¼oz/1 cup)

PUMPKIN
1 serving, raw = 140g
(5oz/1 cup)

Pulses, dairy, nuts and seeds

    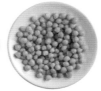

TOFU
1 serving =
110g (4oz/½ cup)

FLAGEOLET BEANS
1 serving, any pulses,
cooked = 90g
(3oz/½ cup)

NUTS & SEEDS
1 serving, any =
40g (1½oz/¼ cup)

FETA CHEESE
1 serving, any soft
cheese = 30g
(1oz/¼ cup)

CHICKPEAS
1 serving, any pulses,
cooked = 90g
(3oz/½ cup)

Wholegrains

**WHOLEWHEAT
BREAD**
1 serving = 1 thin slice
35g (1¼oz)

**WHOLEWHEAT
PASTA**
1 serving, cooked
= 70g (2½oz/½ cup).

QUINOA
1 serving, cooked
= 95g (3½oz/½ cup)

BULGUR WHEAT
1 serving, cooked =
90g (3oz/½ cup)

GRANOLA
1 serving = 75g
(2½oz/½ cup)

BROWN RICE
1 serving, cooked
= 100g (3½oz/½ cup)

You are what you eat

According to the *Upanishads*, the ancient scriptures of India, food is Brahman – the Divine reality. When we eat, we are unified with the environment and with each other. Our food produces the energy that drives our body, but it also shapes our emotions and affects our minds.

Eating with awareness

We live in an age where fast is considered better, and many of us eat hurried meals. Eating in a hurry means that you do not have time to really taste what you are eating, to know when you have eaten enough to satisfy hunger, or to notice the effect that a certain food has on your mood or emotions. On a physical level, hurried eating impairs digestion. On an emotional and psychological level, it separates us from the food we eat. The yogic way is to eat mindfully, being aware of what you are eating and where you are eating it.

ATTITUDE TO FOOD Adopt a balanced, joyful approach to what you eat. Enjoy it, respect it, and be grateful for it. It is a gift of nature. When you cook, your emotions are transferred to the food. Always prepare food with love, allowing your prana to pass to the food and nourish the people you are feeding.

HOW TO EAT Make sure that you are comfortable when you are eating. Always sit down and eat somewhere peaceful. If you eat alone, be silent. If you are with friends or family, avoid arguments and emotional issues. Eat slowly so you really taste the food, chew your food well to prepare it for the stomach, and do not overeat. Keep your awareness on the act of eating.

WHEN TO EAT Eat three meals at regular times each day and always wait until your last meal is digested before eating again. Do not eat if you are not hungry and do not eat a large meal late at night. At bedtime, avoid heavier foods such as dairy and pulses.

WHAT TO EAT Eat unrefined, organic food, preferably locally produced and in season. Do not eat fruit with meals as it may cause bloating and indigestion. Try to eat the lighter food in a meal first. Only sip a little warm water at mealtimes. Liquids dilute the digestive enzymes and impair digestion. Never drink ice-cold water at any time as it is too cold for the body.

The gunas

Sattva This is the quality of purity, truth, light, and love; the higher quality that allows spiritual growth. Sattvic foods promote physical, mental, and spiritual health and they calm the mind. They are fresh, pure, and full of prana. They are also easy to digest and free from chemicals, pesticides, fertilizers, and preservatives. Sattvic foods should make up most of your diet.

Rajas This is the quality of change, activity, and movement. Rajasic foods are stimulating by nature; they include warmed-up or overcooked foods, as well as stale or rotten foods. Used in moderation, they provide the body with vital energy, but in excess, they create imbalance, which leads to restlessness, hyperactivity, and anger.

Tamas This is the quality of dullness, darkness, and inertia. Tamasic foods lead to sluggishness, dullness, and lethargy, and incline the body towards disease. They are difficult to digest and are lacking in prana. Tamasic foods are the ones to be most avoided. They include food that is old, stale, or reheated, leftovers, microwaved food, and canned and frozen food.

Types of food

In the yogic way of eating it is important to keep the three gunas (sattva, rajas, and tamas) in balance. Food is categorized according to the effect it has on each of the gunas. The need to balance the gunas explains why certain foods are not permitted in a yogic diet, even if, to the Western way of thinking, they do not have detrimental physical effects.

	Sattvic foods	Rajasic foods	Tamasic foods
Grains	Freshly prepared grains: rice, wholewheat, oatmeal, barley, millet, unleavened bread	Very hot or salty grain-based foods, e.g. salted porridge; fried bread	Foods made from refined flour: white pasta, pizza, commercial breakfast cereals
Vegetables	Most fresh vegetables and salads	Onions, leeks, radishes, garlic, okra, potatoes, carrots, peppers, chilli peppers, karela (bitter melon)	Mushrooms, potatoes
Fruit	Most fresh fruit and freshly made juices; fresh dates are considered highly sattvic	Unripe fruit, lemons, limes, olives, avocado, tomatoes, bottled juices, canned and sweetened fruit	Canned and sweetened, fermented, and frozen fruit
Sweet foods	Honey; raw, unrefined sugar	White sugar (for its short-term effects), malt syrup, corn syrup, mollasses	White sugar (for its long-term effects), pastries, chocolate, ice cream, jams
Seasoning	Mild spices: cumin, coriander, fennel, fenugreek, cardamom, cinnamon, saffron	Vinegar; hot spices, e.g. chilli, cayenne; mustard; pickles; strong herbs; salt; soya sauce	Pickles and relishes
Pulses	Freshly prepared pulses, e.g. mung beans, aduki beans, black and brown lentils	Very hot or salted pulses	Canned or frozen pulses
Proteins	Nuts (especially almonds); sesame seeds; sunflower seeds; tofu; fresh, pure milk	Eggs, hard cheeses, peanuts, salted nuts, sour cream	Meat; fish; salted nuts; texturized soya protein; milk, pasteurized or homogenized
Drinks	Pure, fresh fruit juice; fresh milk; fresh lassi; herbal teas	Coffee, tea, small amounts of alcohol	Alcohol; soft drinks; milk, pasteurized or homogenized
Fats	Fresh, organic unsalted butter, ghee, and yoghurt; olive oil; sesame oil; flax oil	Salted butter, fried foods	Deep-fried food, lard, margarine

Common concerns about the yogic diet

If you have never tried a vegetarian diet, you are bound to have a lot of questions about it. And if you are a yoga practitioner, or thinking of starting yoga, you may want to understand more about how vegetarianism can support you in your yoga practice.

"Why does the yogic lacto-vegetarian diet include milk and cheese when research shows that these are linked to health problems?"

Traditionally, milk, cream, butter, and yogurt are foods (see pp212–13) and are favoured in a yogic diet. However, with modern dairy farming methods, the degree to which you include dairy in your diet is a matter of personal choice. Cow's milk contains residues of antibiotics and hormones that have been shown to disrupt hormone levels in men and women. Pasteurization and homogenization destroy milk's beneficial bacteria, which makes milk hard to digest and contributes to the rise in dairy allergies and digestive problems.

But the body needs fat; butter and fresh cheese are a good source of nutrients and are not harmful in small amounts. Also, a little dairy can help practically and emotionally if you are trying to switch to a totally vegan diet.

"I practise yoga for at least two hours each day. How will I be able to get enough protein to maintain and build my muscles and strength on a yogic lacto-vegetarian diet?"

It is a myth that you need high levels of protein in order to exercise. Some of the strongest and biggest animals on earth eat a plant-based diet. The protein myth stems from some poor experiments in the 1900s on the protein requirements of rats. Human protein requirements, measured in experiments in the 1950s, indicated that most complex carbohydrates (like those in beans, grains, and vegetables) have all the amino acids required by humans.

Moreover, the once commonly held belief that vegetarians need to eat specific combinations of plant proteins in the same meal to achieve "complete proteins" has been dispelled. We now know that the body has a pool of stored amino acids to complement the amino acids in recently digested food.

In addition, your protein requirements are probably lower than you think. According to the World Health Organization, protein only needs to be five per cent of our total calorie intake. Virtually every single lentil, bean, vegetable, nut, seed, grain, and fruit provides more than five per cent of its calories as protein, and some have much higher levels.

Nor is protein an efficient source of energy. Muscle fatigue sets in when *carbohydrate* stores in the muscles and liver are depleted, so diets that are high in carbohydrates (found in wholegrains, vegetables, and pulses) will prevent fatigue and muscle damage. If you exercise to a particularly strenuous level, then a protein-rich meal or snack, such as sunflower-seed butter on wholegrain toast, after your exercise, will help to prevent depletion of the amino acids in your body.

What this means is that, as long as you are eating enough calories to meet your energy requirements, and not eating a diet full of junk and refined food, then the lacto-vegetarian diet can easily meet all your protein needs.

"I've heard about the acid-alkaline balance. What does this mean and does it have anything to do with vegetarianism?"

Acid is produced in our body for a number of different reasons and generally speaking, the acid-alkaline levels are very precisely controlled by complex biochemical mechanisms. The metabolism of our food and our lifestyle choices can produce a great deal of acid. Whenever we exercise, or even move, our body produces acid. When we get stressed, our acid levels rise. Foods such as animal products, refined grains, fats, and sugar are acid-forming, as are alcohol, coffee, black tea, peanuts, walnuts, preservatives, and hard cheeses.

Too much acid in the body leads to acidosis, which is when acid is deposited in our tissues. This can lead to a multitude of diseases – gout, rheumatism, gall and kidney stones, arteriosclerosis, and heart disease. Migraines and cancers have also been linked to high levels of acidity. And it gets worse. To counteract high levels of acid, the body may take alkaline salts, such as calcium, from the bones. This can lead to osteoporosis.

To combat acidosis, do your yoga practice. Yoga is renowned for being a stress-busting tool. In addition, you should aim for 80 per cent of your food and drink to be alkaline-forming. This is where being a vegetarian comes in. Most plant foods, with the exception of lentils, are alkaline, and even if you eat lentils a few times a week, providing you are following an organic vegetarian diet, then the lentils should not cause you any problems.

"Can diet help my powers of concentration for yoga?"

It is recommended that you follow a Sattvic diet. If your diet is too Rajasic (see pp212–13), you will be restless and unable to sit in meditation. If it is Tamasic (see pp212–13), you will feel too heavy and dull to think with clarity. Avoid stimulants such as tea, coffee, and chocolate.

In addition, we know that the neurons in the brain need essential fats to function properly, so include a small amount of seeds and nuts, and their oils, in your diet. Flax and hemp are particularly good sources. Finally, use rosemary and sage in your cooking or to make infusions. Rosemary is a cerebral stimulant, while sage can clear emotional blocks from the mind and promote calmness and clarity.

The transition towards a yogic diet

This six-week plan will help you to work towards either a lacto-vegetarian or a vegetarian diet. For best results, make the changes gradually and adjust the diet to your own needs. Be aware that

Week 1

☐ Start to take meals at regular times. Eat slowly and chew your food well.

☐ Check your store cupboard and use up or throw away processed foods such as white sugar, biscuits, and tinned sauces.

☐ Shop for organic products only, including in-season fruit and vegetables; wholegrains and pulses; cold-pressed oils for cooking and salad dressings; meat, fish, eggs, and dairy foods.

☐ Reduce meat portions and use more vegetables. Cut out processed meats such as sausages, salami, and burgers.

☐ Cut out all soft drinks such as colas and squashes.

Tip of the week

"Make one vegetarian dish. Read the recipes in this book for ideas."

Week 2

☐ Stop eating all red meat. Replace beef, lamb, and pork with lighter meats such as fish or chicken.

☐ This week, make two vegetarian main meals. Use chickpeas, lentils, and adzuki beans instead of meat in lasagne or casseroles. Try cooking with tofu.

☐ Try different wholegrains with each meal, including brown rice, quinoa, and couscous. Chew them well to avoid bloating and wind.

☐ Try alternatives to coffee made from cereal grains, or reduce the number of cups you drink.

☐ Have three alcohol-free days this week. Try fresh juices diluted with sparkling water.

☐ Visit your local bookshop and choose a vegetarian cook book that inspires you.

"Visit a bookshop and choose an inspiring vegetarian cook book."

Week 3

☐ If you feel ready, cut out all meat except fish. If you miss the texture of meat, use thick slices of aubergine or make nut loaves.

☐ Reduce all your portion sizes of fish and eggs, and increase your portions of vegetables.

☐ Restrict your intake of tea or coffee to no more than two cups a day.

☐ Make three days this week alcohol free.

"Try a vegetarian dish if you are eating out, most restaurants offer a good choice."

you may experience some symptoms of detoxification, like headache, fatigue, or skin problems. If this happens, slow down. You may need six months or longer to achieve your goal.

Week 4

- [ ] Don't eat fish more often than every other day. Use the menu planner (see pp220-1) to plan for fish-free days.

- [ ] If you eat eggs for breakfast, try alternatives such as scrambled tofu with spinach and grilled tomatoes (see p225).

- [ ] Reduce tea and coffee to one cup per day.

- [ ] Don't feel guilty if you haven't reached all your goals. Look at what you are finding most difficult and work out how to make things easier.

"Invite some friends for supper and cook them a vegetarian meal!"

Week 5

- [ ] Reduce your fish intake to two days this week.

- [ ] If you eat eggs every day, try to cut down to every other day.

- [ ] Try using egg alternatives, such as a banana for each egg in cakes or pancakes, or buy egg replacers from your local health food store.

- [ ] If you feel your meals are too light, add a little cold-pressed flaxseed or olive oil to dress your vegetables, or make a tahini dressing (see p235). Make sure you are eating enough whole grains.

- [ ] See if you can avoid drinking alcohol completely, except on special occasions.

- [ ] If family or friends ask you for dinner, let them know that you would prefer not to eat meat or fish – but don't push your ideals upon them.

"Tell family and friends that you are working towards a healthier diet."

Week 6

- [ ] Stop eating all fish and eggs, and enjoy a wide variety of plant foods.

- [ ] Make sure that you are eating the correct number of servings of all the food groups (see the food pyramid p211).

- [ ] Expand your repertoire of recipes by searching in cook books or on the internet.

- [ ] Don't give yourself a strict time limit for changing your diet. Instead of worrying about what you haven't yet achieved, feel proud of the things you have managed to do.

"Congratulations! You've made the change to a healthy yogic diet."

Cooking techniques

Grains and legumes are key to a lacto-vegetarian diet, but people often find them hard to digest. It is important to know how to cook them properly to avoid bloating, gas, or indigestion. Washing and soaking before cooking removes dirt and makes them more digestible. Oils are used in a lacto-vegetarian diet to replace animal fats. Knowing how to store oils correctly to prevent them from turning rancid is essential.

Grains

The key to cooking grains is to measure or weigh them so you know how much water to use. The table below shows you the correct proportion of grains to liquid to produce about 3½ times the volume of the dried grains.

SOAKING AND RINSING Most grains, except for quinoa and millet, will be more digestible if you soak them in cold water before cooking for at least 30 minutes or preferably overnight. Quinoa and millet may be dry-roasted for a few minutes instead. Whether or not you have soaked them first, before cooking rinse the grains in cold water 2–3 times, ideally until the water runs clear.

COOKING Bring the correct amount of water to the boil (see chart), add the grain, and a pinch of salt. Bring back to the boil, reduce the heat, and cover. Simmer until the water has been absorbed. Remove from the heat but leave for a few minutes in the covered pan before serving to dry out the grains.

Cooking times and water volumes

Grain	Uncooked weight	Volume of water	Cooking time	Yield
Barley	200g (7oz)	2½ times	35–40 minutes	560g (1¼lb)
Buckwheat	170g (5¾oz)	2–2½ times	35–40 minutes	600g (1lb 5oz)
Bulgur wheat	175g (6oz)	2 times	35–40 minutes	630g (1lb 6oz)
Couscous	185g (6½oz)	2 times	15 minutes	540g (1lb 3oz)
Millet	195g (6¾oz)	3 times	25–30 minutes	600g (1lb 5oz)
Oats, rolled	115g (4oz)	2¾ times	10 minutes	800g (1¾lb)
Quinoa	180g (6½oz)	2 times	15–20 minutes	800g (1¾lb)
Rice, white basmati	205g (7oz)	2 times	15–20 minutes	650g (1lb 7oz)
Rice, brown basmati	205g (7oz)	2½ times	30–35 minutes	600g (1lb 5oz)
Rice flakes	105g (3½oz)	1¼ times	5–7 minutes	315g (10oz)
Wild rice	180g (6½oz)	4 times	50 minutes	600g (1lb 5oz)

Legumes

Many people have problems digesting beans and pulses. They can cause flatulence and allergies. If you are just starting to add beans to your diet, eat them no more than 1–2 times a week for the first few weeks. After that you may be able to increase your consumption to 3–4 times per week. The most easily digested beans are split mung beans, aduki (adzuki), and black gram beans (urad dal). Following the guidelines below will make beans easier to digest:

SOAKING AND RINSING Always soak beans before cooking. This helps remove the oligosaccharides (a form of carbohydrate) that cause flatulence. Soak for 4 hours or overnight in 3–4 times their volume of water. Soak fava beans and older beans for 24 hours. Rinse before cooking.

COOKING Cook in fresh water. You may need as much as 6 times their volume of water, as some of the water evaporates during cooking. Bring to the boil, partially cover, and simmer until soft. Never eat undercooked beans and do not boil them or add salt or acid ingredients, such as large amounts of lemon juice or tomatoes. This can make them tough and hard to digest.

SERVING Adding ginger, fennel, cumin, or black pepper to cooked beans aids digestion. Traditionally, these spices are sautéed in ghee (clarified butter) or oil, then added to the finished dish.

Oils

Research shows that trans fats contribute more than unsaturated fats to cardiovascular disease. Trans fats are formed when oils are exposed to heat and air, so it is vital to know how to store oils and which to use for cooking.

STORING Always store oils in a dark place and choose oils that are packaged in dark glass or metal containers. Avoid those that are sold in clear plastic bottles. Stable oils – those that are not damaged when exposed to high temperatures, such as ghee and olive oil – can be stored in a dark cupboard. Cold-pressed oils, such as avocado, flaxseed, safflower, and sunflower oils, are very unstable and should be kept in the refrigerator.

COOKING For cooking at high temperatures, especially above 160°C/325°F/Gas 3 as when baking in the oven, only use the most stable oils. Choose from organic ghee, organic sesame oil, palm kernel oil, or coconut oil. You can sauté food at moderate temperatures using olive oil. Never use the unstable, cold-pressed oils mentioned above for cooking.

A Week's Menu

The week's menu plan given below will help to ease your transition to a vegetarian diet. For each day of the week there is a suggested breakfast, lunch, and dinner, as well as some snacks and

	Monday	Tuesday	Wednesday
Breakfast	Vanilla quinoa cereal p222, served with maple syrup	Spiced oat or millet porridge p224	Morning energy shake p225
Lunch	Soba noodles with stir-fry vegetables and tofu p231	Basic vegetable soup p242, Pea and quinoa salad p227	Roasted Tuscan wraps p233, served with a green salad, Parsley and nut or seed dressing p235
Dinner	Stuffed butternut squash with sage p238, Mediterranean spinach p236	Kicharee p240, Chapati p245	Pumpkin, courgette, and sweet potato stew with bulghur wheat p241
Snacks and sweet treats	Dry-roasted chickpeas with spice p248	Miso and hazelnut spread p249, with oat cakes	Fresh organic fruit, a mix of sesame and sunflower seeds

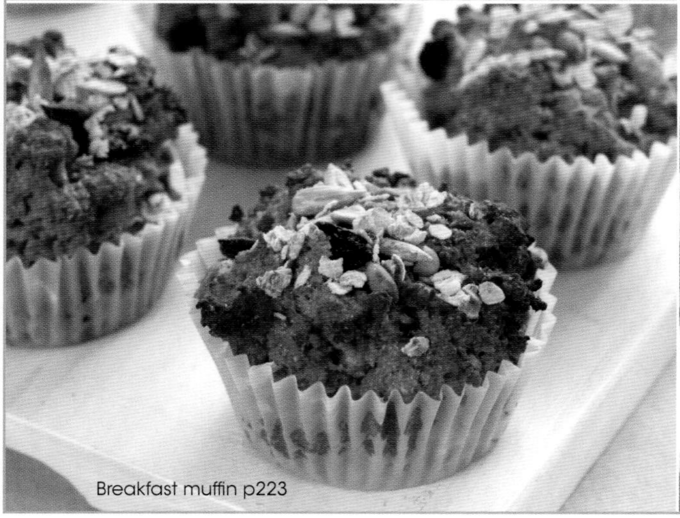

Breakfast muffin p223

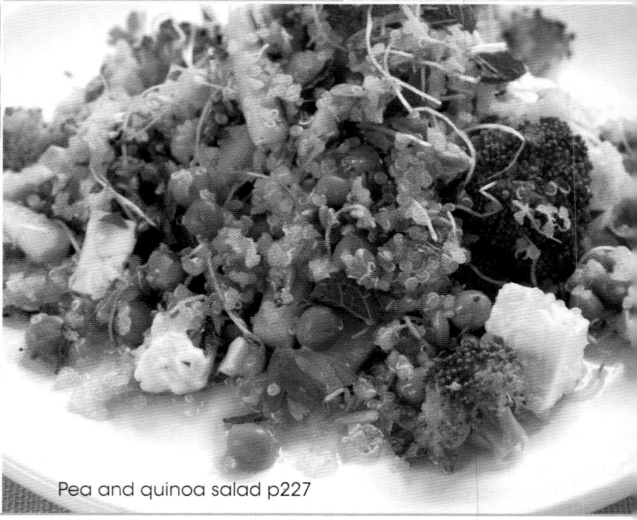

Pea and quinoa salad p227

sweet treats. All the recipes are found in this chapter. The plan has been designed for variety and interest, but you should feel free to make substitutions to suit your own taste.

Thursday	Friday	Saturday	Sunday
Scrambled tofu and vegetables p225, served with toasted organic rye bread	Crispy granola p224, served with organic natural yogurt	Buckwheat banana pancakes p225, served with maple syrup	Fresh fruit salad, Breakfast muffin p223
Roasted vegetables and chickpeas with couscous p226, Buckwheat pitta bread p244, served with a green salad	Sweet cinnamon dhal p228, Brown basmati rice p218, Chapati p245, served with steamed green beans	Millet burgers p231, Walnut coleslaw p234, Gomasio p237, served with a green salad, Fruit crumble p247	Vegetable coconut curry p229, Brown basmati rice p218, Sweet sesame carrots p236, Coriander and coconut chutney p237
Barley risotto p243	Pasta with tofu pesto p241, served with a green salad	Tomato, red lentil, and barley soup p239	Basic vegetable soup p242, Pumpkin soda bread p244
Fresh organic fruit	Dried raisins, a mix of sesame and sunflower seeds	Fresh organic fruit, a mix of sesame and sunflower seeds	Chocolate and silken tofu mousse p246

Tomato, red lentil, and barley soup p239

Fruit crumble p247

Breakfast

In our fast-paced world, breakfast all too often consists of a snatched coffee and croissant or a processed high-sugar cereal. Instead, start your day as you mean to go on: take at least 15 minutes to eat slowly and in a relaxed environment, enjoying freshly prepared wholegrains that sustain your mood and energy.

Home-made muesli

There are many proprietary mueslis available, but it's also fun to make your own – and far more economical.

Serves 4

Choose a total of 5 tbsp from any of the following grains:
barley flakes
oat flakes
wheat flakes
millet flakes *
rice flakes *
quinoa flakes *
buckwheat flakes *

* For a gluten-free diet, choose ingredients marked with an asterisk.

1. Place the mixed flakes into a bowl and add either 1 tbsp of desiccated coconut or 1 tbsp of mixed ground seeds (sunflower, linseeds, and sesame). You can also add 1 tbsp of raisins or dried, chopped dates.
2. Add filtered water or your choice of milk and leave to soak for at least 10 minutes before eating. If you have time, it is even better to soak the flakes overnight in water, since soaking makes them more easily digested.
3. It is a good idea to make a larger batch of these mixed flakes and store them in an airtight container, adding the seeds, coconut, or dried fruit just as you are about to serve each day. Ground seeds should be stored in the refrigerator to avoid oxidation.

Vanilla quinoa cereal

Quinoa is a good source of protein and calcium, giving you a nutrient-packed start while being light on the stomach.

Serves 4

200g (7oz) quinoa
500ml (16fl oz) almond milk (see p249)
1 vanilla pod, split
a grating of nutmeg
2 tbsp maple syrup

1. Place the quinoa in a sieve over the sink and rinse thoroughly under cold running water until the water runs clear.
2. Put the rinsed quinoa into a medium-sized saucepan and cover with 250ml (8fl oz) cold, filtered water. Bring to the boil over a medium heat, then cover with a tight-fitting lid, reduce the heat, and simmer for about 15 minutes, stirring frequently, or until the quinoa is light, fluffy, and cooked.
3. Put the almond milk, split vanilla pod, and a grating of nutmeg into a small saucepan, place over a low heat and warm gently.
4. When you are ready to serve, mix the warm spiced milk into the cooked quinoa and stir well. Serve with maple syrup.

Breakfast muffins

To make these muffins even healthier, replace 25g (scant 1oz)
flour with oat bran, which helps to reduce cholesterol levels.

Makes 6

150g (5½oz) plain wholemeal flour, sifted
25g (scant 1oz) rolled porridge oats
2 tsp baking powder
½ tsp mixed spice
½ tsp cinnamon
50g (1¾oz) raisins
50g (1¾oz) dried apricots, chopped
25g (scant 1oz) pumpkin seeds
25g (scant 1oz) soft brown sugar
3 tbsp olive oil
1 medium banana, mashed
1 medium carrot, coarsely grated
3 tbsp cow's or soya milk

To decorate

handful of mixed sunflower and
pumpkin seeds
handful of rolled porridge oats

1. Preheat the oven to 190°C (375°F/Gas 5). Put 6 muffin cases on a lightly oiled baking tray.

2. Combine the dry ingredients in a large bowl and set aside. In another bowl, combine the remaining ingredients thoroughly. Add to the dry ingredients and stir until just combined.

3. Spoon the mixture into the prepared muffin cases.

4. Sprinkle with sunflower and pumpkin seeds and oats. Bake for 20–30 minutes or until a toothpick inserted into the middle of a muffin comes out clean.

5. Allow the muffins to cool in the tray for 5 minutes, then remove and place on a wire rack to cool completely. They are delicious served with organic butter, jam, or cottage cheese.

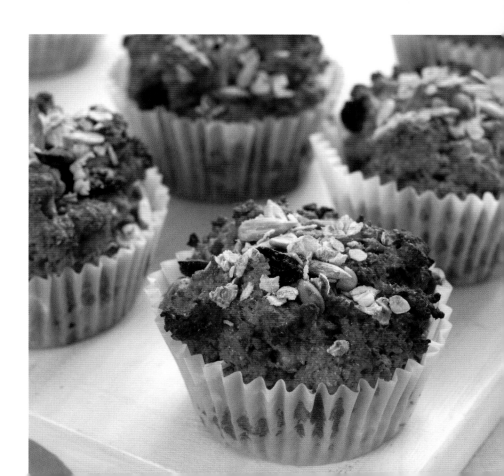

Dried fruit compôte

In summer, fresh fruit can be used for a healthy fruit salad – but
in winter, a warm compôte of dried fruit may be more appealing.

Serves 4
200g (7oz) dried apricots
100g (3½oz) prunes
100g (3½oz) dried pears
3 cloves
1 cinnamon stick
2 tbsp freshly squeezed orange juice

1. Place the dried fruit in a bowl with the spices, orange juice, and 600ml (1 pint) filtered water, and leave to soak overnight.

2. The next morning, pour the mixture into a pan and bring to the boil. Reduce the heat, partially cover the pan, and simmer for 30 minutes. Remove the spices and serve.

Spiced oat or millet porridge

Millet flakes cook as quickly as oats, and the porridge tends to be
smoother. The flavour is less strong, so using the spices is important.

Serves 4
200g (7oz) rolled oats or millet flakes
4 tbsp raisins
½ tsp ground cardamom
½ tsp ground ginger
To serve
160ml (5½fl oz) organic cow's or soya milk
2 tbsp maple syrup or honey (optional)
freshly grated nutmeg, to taste

1. In a medium-sized saucepan over a medium heat, bring 1.5 litres (2½ pints) filtered water to the boil. Pour in the oats or millet, raisins, and spices, stirring continually as you do so.

2. Reduce the heat and simmer gently, stirring occasionally, until the porridge reaches a creamy consistency (7–10 minutes).

3. Serve in bowls and add milk and grated nutmeg to taste. If a sweeter porridge is desired, add some honey or maple syrup.

Crispy granola

This is lovely served with fresh yogurt or simply as an alternative
to home-made muesli (see p222).

Serves 4
3 tbsp maple syrup
a few drops of vanilla extract
1 tbsp ground cinnamon
200g (7oz) rolled oats
75g (2½oz) oat bran
75g (2½oz) sunflower seeds
60g (2oz) pumpkin seeds
150g (5½oz) raisins

1. Preheat the oven to 160°C (325°F/Gas 3).

2. Mix the maple syrup, vanilla extract, and cinnamon with 3 tbsp hot water.

3. Mix the oats, oat bran, sunflower seeds, and pumpkin seeds together in a large mixing bowl. Stir in the maple syrup solution and mix well.

4. Spread the mixture onto two lightly oiled baking trays and bake in the oven, stirring occasionally for 20–25 minutes until golden. Add the raisins and bake for a further 5 minutes. Leave to cool and store in an airtight container.

Buckwheat banana pancakes

These pancakes are a great treat for a weekend breakfast, and
are particularly tasty served with maple syrup.

Serves 4

75g (2½oz) buckwheat flour
¼ tsp ground allspice
¼ tsp ground cinnamon
½ tsp baking powder
pinch sea salt
120ml (4fl oz) almond milk (enough
to form a smooth batter, see p249 for
recipe)
1 small banana, sliced
small handful fresh blueberries
1 tsp sunflower oil
maple syrup, to serve

1. Sift together the flour, allspice, cinnamon, baking powder, and sea salt into a large bowl, and mix well.

2. Gradually pour in the almond milk and beat until the mixture has become a smooth liquid. Stir in the sliced banana and blueberries.

3. Place a frying pan over a medium–high heat, add the oil, and swirl the pan to ensure the whole surface is lightly coated in oil.

4. Pour a small ladleful of the batter into the pan to make a small pancake. Leave for a few minutes and when small air bubbles appear on the surface of the pancake, flip and cook on the other side until golden brown. Repeat with the rest of the batter to make about 8 pancakes. Serve drizzled with maple syrup.

Scrambled tofu and vegetables

This is a great substitute for scrambled eggs; the tofu absorbs all
the flavours, so it's very tasty.

Serves 4

2 tsp olive oil or ghee (clarified butter)
½ tsp turmeric
handful finely chopped asparagus,
broccoli, or courgette
2 tomatoes, peeled and diced
300g (10oz) plain tofu, cut into chunks
and mashed until small and crumbled
handful of finely chopped parsley
pinch of rock salt and pepper, to taste

1. Heat the oil or ghee in a pan on a medium heat and sauté the turmeric and vegetables with a splash of water for about 2 minutes.

2. Add the tofu and herbs and sauté for a further 4–6 minutes, until the flavours mingle and the mixture is heated through.

3. Add salt and pepper to taste, and serve.

Morning energy shake

This is a good digestive aid and a great source of iron.
It packs a powerful energy punch for those very busy days.

Serves 4

8 large dried dates
8 dried unsulphured apricots
240ml (8fl oz) organic plain yogurt
720ml (24fl oz) organic cow's, goat's,
or soya milk

1. Place the dried fruit in a bowl, cover with 500ml (16fl oz) filtered water, and leave to soak overnight.

2. In the morning, pour the soaked dried fruit and its water, the yogurt, and milk into a blender and whizz until smooth. Add more milk to taste.

3. For a more spicy flavour, add ½ tsp ground ginger, or some ground cardamom for a sweeter taste.

Lunch

While lunch should form the main meal of the day, many people with busy work schedules have less time for lunch and more for dinner. However, it should still be possible to include at least one cooked grain, one or more cooked vegetables, and, depending on your digestion and the season, a small serving of raw vegetables in the form of a salad. Extra protein can be provided by including tofu or beans, a small serving of soft cheese, or a dressing or condiment made with nuts or seeds.

Roasted vegetables and chickpeas with couscous

Couscous, made from semolina wheat, is an easy grain to prepare.
You can vary the vegetables; adjust the cooking time as necessary.

Serves 4

125g (4½oz) dried chickpeas, soaked overnight in 500ml (16fl oz) filtered water
150g (5½oz) parsnips
150g (5½oz) sweet potatoes
150g (5½oz) celeriac
150g (5½oz) carrots
150g (5½oz) beetroot
1 tsp dried mixed herbs
2 tsp caraway seeds
4 tbsp sesame oil
freshly ground black pepper and a pinch of salt
125g (4½oz) couscous, rinsed several times in cold water
drizzle of lemon juice and olive oil
chapatis (see p245)

1. Drain the chickpeas after soaking and place in a pan with 500ml (16fl oz) water. Bring to the boil, cook uncovered for 20 minutes, and then partially cover and cook for another 1–1½ hours until tender. Drain and set aside to cool.

2. Preheat the oven to 180°C (350°F/Gas 4).

3. Cut all the root vegetables into evenly sized chunks and place them in a large baking tray, together with the herbs and caraway seeds. Toss with the sesame oil and season with black pepper and a pinch of salt.

4. Roast for about 1 hour, turning occasionally to prevent burning.

5. When the vegetables are almost cooked, add the rinsed and drained chickpeas and return to the oven for about 10 minutes.

6. Meanwhile, prepare the rinsed couscous. Place it in a bowl, cover with 250ml (8fl oz) hot, filtered water, and leave to soak for 10 minutes.

7. To serve, separate the grains of couscous with a fork and divide between 4 dinner plates. Add the vegetables and drizzle with a little lemon juice and olive oil to taste.

8. Serve with flat breads such as chapatis.

Pea and quinoa salad

Technically a fruit, quinoa is a highly nutritious food. It has a high protein and calcium content, and is a good source of iron and B vitamins.

Serves 4

175g (6oz) quinoa

400g (14oz) tenderstem broccoli, cut into florets

175g (6oz) fresh peas or sugar snap peas

½ large cucumber, cut into thin matchsticks

100g (3½oz) green olives, chopped (optional)

200g (7oz) organic goat's cheese, crumbled

45g (1½oz) mixed seeds or pine nuts, toasted

2 tbsp flat-leaf parsley, chopped

2 tbsp fresh mint, chopped

3 tbsp extra virgin olive oil

2 tbsp pumpkin seed oil

½ lemon, juice only

salt and freshly ground black pepper

45g (1½oz) alfalfa or watercress

1. Place the quinoa into a dry saucepan over a medium heat and stir to lightly toast the grains. Add 900ml (1½ pints) cold, filtered water, bring to the boil, reduce the heat and simmer for about 15 minutes or until all the water has been absorbed and the grains are tender. Tip the quinoa onto a large plate to cool quickly.

2. Steam the broccoli and peas or sugar snaps until tender, then tip them into a sieve and place them under running cold water to cool them quickly and stop them cooking further. Put the cooled, cooked quinoa and cooked broccoli and peas or sugar snaps into a large bowl and add the rest of the ingredients (except the oils, lemon juice, and alfalfa sprouts) and mix well.

3. For the dressing, mix the olive oil, pumpkin oil, and lemon juice and season to taste.

4. When you are ready to serve, pour over the dressing, and scatter with the alfalfa sprouts or watercress.

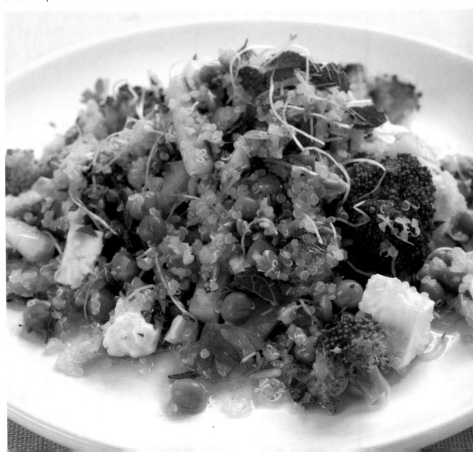

Vegetarian shepherd's pie

The original meat version is better known, but shepherd's pie is easily translated into a tasty and nutritious vegetarian dish.

Serves 4

For the vegetable and lentil base
100g (3½oz) brown lentils
1 tbsp olive oil
200g (7oz) carrots, finely sliced
200g (7oz) parsnips, finely sliced
3–4 celery sticks, sliced
1 bay leaf
225g (8oz) fresh tomatoes, skinned and chopped
sprig of rosemary, finely chopped
1 tsp dried oregano
1 tbsp tamari sauce
salt and freshly ground black pepper

For the potato mash
700g (1lb 9oz) potatoes, peeled and roughly chopped
40g (1¼oz) organic butter
3 tbsp olive oil
3–5 tbsp organic cow's or soya milk
75g (2½oz) organic cheddar cheese, grated (optional)
rocket and carrot, to serve

1. Rinse the lentils until the water runs clear, then cook in 4 times their volume of water until they are tender (about 1 hour).

2. Preheat the oven to 200°C (400°F/Gas 6).

3. Heat the olive oil in a pan and sauté the carrots, parsnips, and celery until almost tender. Add a little water and the bay leaf, then cover and cook until the carrots are tender. Add the lentils, tomatoes, rosemary, and dried oregano and cook for a few more minutes. Season to taste with tamari sauce and salt and pepper.

4. Cook the potatoes in boiling, salted water. When tender, drain and mash with the butter, olive oil, and milk to obtain creamy (not sloppy) mashed potatoes. Season to taste.

5. Spoon the vegetables and lentil mixture into an ovenproof dish, remove the bay leaf and top with the mashed potato. If desired, sprinkle over the grated cheese. Bake for 30–40 minutes, until the top is nicely browned. Serve with a salad of rocket and carrot.

Sweet cinnamon dhal

Traditionally, split mung beans are used in dhal dishes, but this recipe uses red lentils, which are more readily available.

Serves 4

1 tbsp ghee (clarified butter) or sesame oil
½ tsp black mustard seeds
½ tsp turmeric
½ tsp ground fennel or fennel seeds
½ tsp ground cinnamon
1 tsp ground coriander
275g (9¾oz) red lentils, soaked in filtered water for 30 minutes
¾ tsp salt
2 tsp lemon juice
1 tsp maple syrup
brown rice, chapatis (see p245), and your choice of vegetables

1. Heat the ghee or sesame oil in a large saucepan and add the black mustard seeds. When they pop, add all the remaining spices and cook for several minutes, stirring continually, to release their aromas.

2. Drain the lentils, add to the pan with 750ml (1¼ pints) filtered water, and bring to the boil. Reduce the heat, partially cover, and simmer for 25–30 minutes, stirring occasionally, until the mixture is thick and the lentils are soft.

3. To give a more creamy texture, blend half of the cooked dhal in a blender or food processor, return to the pan and stir well. If the mixture is too thick, add an additional splash of water. Add the salt, lemon juice, and maple syrup to taste and serve with brown rice, chapatis, and vegetables.

Vegetable coconut curry

This delicious curry is mild and sweet in flavour. It involves a little preparation the night before but is quick to make on the day.

Serves 4

150g (5½oz) unsweetened organic desiccated coconut

125g (4½oz) dried chickpeas, soaked overnight in 500ml (16fl oz) water

3 tsp cumin seeds

1 tsp coriander seeds

½ tsp fennel seeds

2 tbsp ghee (clarified butter)

3 cardamom pods, seeds only

½ tsp ground cinnamon

pinch ground cloves

½ tsp ground ginger

25g (1oz) fresh root ginger, peeled and grated

2 large vine-ripened tomatoes, skinned, seeded, and roughly chopped

200g (7oz) butternut squash, cut into cubes, or 1 large sweet potato, cut into cubes

2 carrots, roughly chopped

100g (3½oz) fresh spinach, stalks removed, roughly chopped

squeeze of fresh lime juice, or to taste

1 tbsp maple syrup

salt and freshly ground black pepper

4 tbsp fresh coriander, roughly chopped

brown basmati rice, sweet sesame carrots (see p236), and chapatis (see p245) to serve

1. To make the coconut milk, place the desiccated coconut into a bowl and pour 20fl oz (600ml) boiling, filtered water over it. Stir to combine and leave to soak for 10 minutes, then whizz in a blender on high for 1 minute. Leave for a further 10 minutes and then pass through a sieve into a bowl, using the back of a spoon to squeeze out all the excess moisture. Discard the coconut remaining in the sieve.

2. Drain the soaked chickpeas and rinse under cold running water. Tip them into a medium-sized saucepan, cover with 360ml (12fl oz) cold water, and bring to the boil. Cover with a lid, reduce the heat to a simmer, and cook for 1½–2 hours or until tender and then drain.

3. In a large pan, dry fry the cumin, coriander, and fennel seeds over a medium heat for about 1 minute or until fragrant. Tip into a mortar and pestle and grind to a powder with the rest of the spices. Heat the ghee in the pan, add the ground spices and grated ginger, and fry over a gentle heat for 1–2 minutes. Add the tomatoes, stir well, and cook for another minute.

4. Add the prepared coconut milk to the tomato and spice mix and simmer over a medium heat for 5 minutes or until the sauce has thickened slightly.

5. Meanwhile, in a separate pan, steam the butternut squash or sweet potato cubes and carrots for 6–8 minutes or until just tender. Add the steamed vegetables to the tomato, coconut, and spice mix, then add the spinach, cooked chickpeas, lime juice, and maple syrup. Season well to taste, then simmer for 2–3 minutes. Loosen with a little water if the sauce is too thick, stir in the chopped coriander, and serve. Brown basmati rice, sweet sesame carrots, and chapatis make excellent accompaniments.

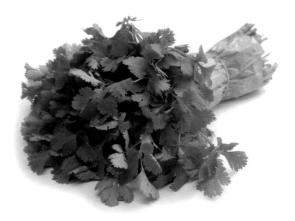

CORIANDER
Coriander not only adds a pleasant, fresh flavour, it is also full of nutrients and is thought to aid digestion.

Tofu kebabs with saffron rice

Rich in protein, B vitamins, and calcium, tofu takes on the
flavours of a marinade to make a delicious basis for a meal.

Serves 4

For the kebabs

3 tbsp tamari sauce

zest of 1 orange and the juice of half of it

1 tsp grated fresh root ginger

1 tbsp olive oil

½ tsp turmeric

small handful of fresh coriander leaves, chopped

¾ tsp salt and freshly ground black pepper

500g (1lb 2oz) firm tofu, cut into large cubes

2 courgettes, sliced

8 cherry tomatoes

For the rice

pinch of saffron strands

1 tsp cumin seeds

250g (9oz) basmati rice, washed until the water runs clear

½ tsp rock salt

carrot and raisin salad (see p234) and chapatis (see p245)

1. Make the marinade by mixing the tamari sauce, orange zest, orange juice, ginger, olive oil, turmeric, and chopped coriander. Season with salt and freshly ground black pepper. Pour the marinade over the tofu cubes, cover, and refrigerate for 2 hours.

2. Thread the tofu cubes onto 8 wooden kebab sticks, alternating them with the courgette slices and tomatoes. Baste the courgettes and tomatoes with any remaining marinade.

3. Preheat the grill.

4. To make the rice, dry roast the saffron and cumin in a heavy-bottomed, medium-sized saucepan for 2–3 minutes. Add the rice, 750ml (1¼ pints) filtered water, and rock salt. Bring to the boil, cover, and reduce the heat to low. Cook for about 10 minutes, until all the water has been absorbed and the rice grains are soft.

5. While the rice is cooking, arrange the kebabs on the grill pan and cook for 8–10 minutes, turning frequently and basting with the marinade.

6. Serve the kebabs with the saffron rice, carrot and raisin salad, and chapatis or other flat bread.

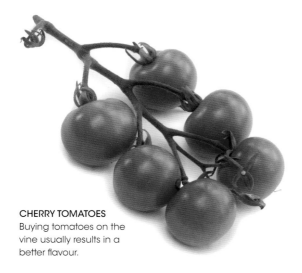

CHERRY TOMATOES
Buying tomatoes on the
vine usually results in a
better flavour.

Soba noodles with stir-fry vegetables and tofu

As they are made from buckwheat, soba noodles are a good alternative for those on a gluten-free diet, and are quick to cook.

Serves 4

4 tbsp tamari

4 tbsp lemon juice

1 tsp grated root ginger

handful of fresh coriander, chopped, plus extra for garnish

freshly ground black pepper

500g (1lb 2oz) tofu, finely cubed

250g (9oz) soba noodles, thick rice noodles, or udon noodles

sesame oil, for frying

about 600g (1lb 5oz) mixed vegetables such as red and green peppers, carrots, broccoli, courgettes, and bean sprouts

toasted sesame seeds and fresh coriander, to garnish

1. Mix the tamari, lemon juice, ginger, and coriander in a bowl and season with black pepper. Toss the tofu in the marinade and leave for 15–30 minutes.

2. Meanwhile, slice the vegetables into uniformly sized pieces.

3. Cook the noodles according to the packet instructions, in a large pan of boiling water. Drain, rinse, and set aside.

4. Heat a heavy pan or wok and brush lightly with sesame oil. Keep the heat high and add all the vegetables except the bean sprouts, if using. Add 2 tbsp water and toss from side to side gently with a wooden spoon for about 3 minutes. Add the tofu and its marinade and fry for a further 3 minutes. Finally, add the bean sprouts and cooked noodles and cook for 1–2 minutes more until the noodles are warm. Serve immediately, garnished with sesame seeds and some fresh coriander.

Millet burgers

Millet is a gluten-free grain, easy to digest and with a cooling and soothing effect on the digestive system.

Makes about 4 large burgers

200g (7oz) millet

4 tbsp fresh herbs (sage, basil, or parsley), chopped

125g (4½oz) courgettes, grated

75g (2½oz) roasted and ground almonds or sunflower seeds

1 tbsp olive or sesame oil

1 tsp turmeric

1–2 tbsp wholegrain flour (if on a gluten-free diet, substitute with buckwheat or soya flour)

salt and freshly ground black pepper

1. Bring 800ml (1½ pints) filtered water to the boil, add the millet, stir well, and bring to the boil again. Reduce the heat, cover, and simmer for about 30 minutes or until the millet is soft and all the liquid has been absorbed. Leave to cool.

2. When the millet is cold, mash with the chopped herbs. Add the grated courgette, ground almonds or sunflower seeds, oil, turmeric, and 1 tbsp of the flour. Season generously and stir well to make a thick mixture.

3. Shape the mixture into 4 burger shapes, adding the remaining flour if the consistency feels too wet – handle with care as the mixture has a tendency to crumble. To help retain the shape of the burgers during cooking, refrigerate for 30 minutes.

4. Preheat the oven to 180°C (350°F/Gas 4).

5. Remove the burgers from the refrigerator and bake in the oven for 30 minutes until heated through and golden. Alternatively, you can sauté them in a lightly oiled or non-stick pan, pressing down with a spatula and turning over with care when golden brown.

Yam pie with a crunchy nutty crust

This recipe uses amaranth flour, which is available in some health shops and also online from suppliers of gluten-free products.

Serves 4

For the crust

75g (2½oz) ground sunflower seeds

75g (2½oz) ground almonds

75g (2½oz) amaranth flour (if unavailable, use wholewheat or rye flour)

¾ tsp cinnamon

pinch of rock salt

3 tbsp sesame oil

1½ tbsp apple juice

For the filling

3 medium yams, chopped into 1cm (½in) chunks (if yams are not available use 5 medium-sized sweet potatoes)

1 tsp ghee (clarified butter) or sesame oil

3 celery sticks, sliced

15g (½oz) butter

1 tbsp soya milk

1 tbsp arrowroot powder

½ tsp cinnamon

pinch each of ground nutmeg, ground allspice and ground cloves

1. Preheat the oven to 180°C (350°F/Gas 4).

2. To make the crust, mix all the dry ingredients together thoroughly. Mix the sesame oil and apple juice together and slowly add them to the dry ingredients. Mix with a fork until a crumbly texture is formed.

3. Press the mixture into an oiled 23cm (9in) pie dish to make a 5mm (¼in) layer on the bottom and sides of the dish. Reserve 1–2 tbsp of the crust mixture for the top of the pie.

4. Place the crust in the oven and bake for 4–5 minutes, then remove immediately to cool.

5. To make the filling, steam the yams or sweet potatoes until very tender (about 10–15 minutes).

6. Heat the ghee or oil and sauté the celery until soft.

7. Mash the yams with the butter, and mix with the celery and remaining ingredients. Place the yam mixture in the cooled piecrust and smooth the top with a knife.

8. Sprinkle with the reserved crust mixture and bake in the oven at 180°C (350°F/Gas 4) for 50–60 minutes until firm and browned.

9. Cool for at least 5 minutes before slicing. Serve with a green vegetable or salad and a dish of peas or beans if desired.

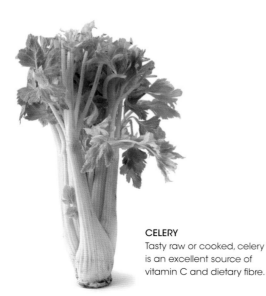

CELERY
Tasty raw or cooked, celery is an excellent source of vitamin C and dietary fibre.

Roasted Tuscan wraps

These adaptable wraps contain good-quality protein, and are ideal for a healthy packed lunch.

Serves 4

2 large courgettes, halved lengthways and de-seeded
4 red peppers, cut in half and de-seeded
2 tbsp sesame oil
2 tsp dried oregano
2 tsp dried rosemary
salt and freshly ground black pepper
75g (2½oz) toasted pine nuts
200g (7oz) soft goat's cheese
4 organic ready-made wraps, or 8 small chapatis (see p245), warmed
8 large handfuls of watercress

1. Preheat the oven to 180°C (350°F/Gas 4). Slice the courgettes across into chunky half moons, place them in a baking tray with the peppers, oil, and herbs, and season to taste. Place on the middle shelf of the oven and roast for 30 minutes or until the skin of the peppers has begun to brown.

2. Remove the vegetables from the oven, setting the courgettes aside to cool. To loosen the skins, place the peppers in a plastic bag and leave until they are cool enough to handle. Remove the skins and slice the flesh into thick strips.

3. In a dry pan over a moderate heat, toast the pine nuts for about 3 minutes, or until just golden.

4. Spread a layer of goat's cheese on each warmed wrap or chapati and divide the peppers, courgettes, watercress, and pine nuts between them. Wrap tightly and serve straight away or store in a cool place until required.

CALIFORNIAN WRAP Spread wraps or chapatis (see p245) with mashed avocado. Layer with tomato slices, spinach, and sprouted mung beans, then finish with a pinch of black pepper.

MIDDLE EASTERN WRAP Use hummus as the base; add beetroot slices and plenty of fresh rocket.

TEMPEH WRAP Use 50g (1¾oz) tempeh (fermented soya) per person. Steam the tempeh and cut into slices. Spread avocado slices on a chapati and add the tempeh, a handful of spinach, slices of tomato, and some grated carrot to add crunch.

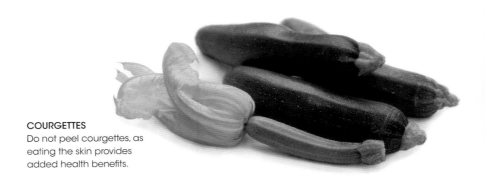

COURGETTES
Do not peel courgettes, as eating the skin provides added health benefits.

Salads and dressings

Raw foods are an important source of prana (see p178) and enzymes. Salads are a great way to include raw vegetables, leaves, and herbs in meals, but as they are hard to digest they are best eaten as a side dish at lunchtime when digestion is at its strongest.

Walnut coleslaw

Home-made coleslaw is a revelation compared to the shop-bought version, and is quick to make.

Serves 4

50g (2oz) shelled walnuts, chopped
2 tbsp pine nuts
1 tbsp sesame seeds
1 tbsp sunflower seeds
¼ large red cabbage, finely shredded
1 large carrot, peeled and grated
50g (2oz) sultanas (optional)
4 tbsp plain natural yogurt
juice of half a lime
3 tbsp walnut oil
2 tsp maple syrup
¼ tsp salt
freshly ground black pepper to taste
3 tbsp fresh mint, coriander, or basil, chopped, plus a few whole leaves, to garnish

1. Put the walnuts, pine nuts, sesame and sunflower seeds in a sauté pan and dry fry them over a medium heat, shaking frequently, for about 1 minute, or until lightly toasted and fragrant.
2. Place the shredded cabbage, carrot, sultanas, toasted walnuts, pine nuts, sesame seeds, and sunflower seeds into a large bowl and mix well.
3. For the dressing, mix the natural yogurt, lime juice, walnut oil, maple syrup, salt and pepper and whisk to combine.
4. Pour the dressing over the cabbage, add the herbs, and combine well.
5. Scatter with the whole mint, coriander, or basil leaves before serving.

Carrot and raisin salad

In this recipe, the sweetness of the carrots and raisins is tempered with spices and lemon juice.

Serves 4

40g (1¼oz) raisins
2 tbsp sesame oil
½ tsp cumin seeds
½ tsp black mustard seeds
pinch of ground coriander
2 medium carrots, grated
1 tbsp fresh lemon juice
½ tsp honey
2 tbsp fresh coriander and
1 tsp sesame seeds, to garnish

1. Soak the raisins in 500ml (16fl oz) hot, filtered water for 10 minutes to make them easier to digest.
2. Heat 1 tbsp sesame oil in a small pan and add the cumin and black mustard seeds. When they start to pop, add the coriander and cook for 1 minute, stirring constantly.
3. Place the soaked raisins, cooked seeds, grated carrots, lemon juice, and honey in a bowl with the remaining sesame oil. Mix well, garnish with coriander and sesame seeds, and serve.

Basic lemon and olive oil dressing

Many salad dressings are very high in preservatives and most contain vinegar, which is avoided on the yogic diet.

Serves 4

75ml (2½fl oz) freshly squeezed lemon juice (about 2 lemons)

75–120ml (2½–4fl oz) extra virgin olive oil

2 tsp honey (optional)

salt and pepper to taste

1. Whisk together all the ingredients in a small bowl, using a fork or chef's hand whisk.

2. For added flavour and variety, you could whisk in some fresh or dried herbs such as tarragon, rosemary, sage, parsley, or oregano.

Tahini dressing

This dressing goes particularly well with bitter leaves – try it with dandelion leaves or watercress.

Serves 4

2 heaped tsp tahini (sesame paste)

4 tsp cold-pressed organic sesame or olive oil

2 tsp lemon juice

freshly ground black pepper (optional)

1. With a fork, mix all the ingredients together in a cup, adding 4 tsp filtered water.

2. Use immediately, drizzling over salad leaves.

Parsley and nut or seed dressing

Parsley is a good source of Vitamin C and beta-carotene, which the body converts into Vitamin A.

Serves 4

1 large bunch fresh parsley

60g (2oz) pumpkin seeds or hazelnuts

1 tsp salt

75ml (2½fl oz) lemon juice

2 tbsp sunflower oil

1. Wash and chop the parsley.

2. Chop the pumpkin seeds or hazelnuts.

3. Put all the ingredients in a blender with 250ml (8fl oz) filtered water and blend until a smooth consistency is reached.

HAZELNUTS
These are a useful source of vitamins B and E.

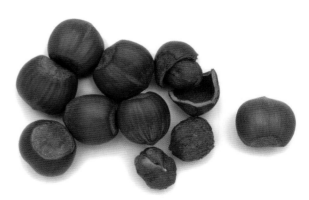

Vegetables and condiments

Vegetables are not only an excellent source of vitamins and minerals, but also contain phytonutrients that are thought to protect against cancer. They have an alkalizing effect on the body, so should form a large part of everyone's diet. In addition to the vegetables in your main dish, always try to include some cooked vegetables as a side dish.

Mediterranean spinach

This traditional recipe from the Mediterranean region offers fresh, sharp flavours and requires only minimal preparation.

Serves 4

60ml (2fl oz) olive oil
75g (2½oz) pine nuts
1kg (2¼lb) young spinach, washed and tough stalks removed
salt and freshly ground black pepper
50g (1¾oz) currants
1 tbsp lemon juice
⅛ tsp ground nutmeg
⅛ tsp ground cinnamon

1. Heat the olive oil in a large sauté pan. Add the pine nuts and sauté over low heat, stirring continuously, until they are lightly browned.

2. Add the washed spinach and season with a little salt and pepper. Stir, cover, and cook for about 2–3 minutes, until the spinach has wilted. If necessary, drain any excess moisture from the pan.

3. Stir in the currants, lemon juice, nutmeg, and cinnamon and serve the spinach immediately.

Sweet sesame carrots

Carrots are high in natural sugar. This recipe capitalizes on that and adds some spice to the sweetness.

Serves 4

1 tsp sesame oil
2 tsp sunflower oil
1 tsp yellow or black mustard seeds
½ tsp turmeric
1 tsp ground coriander
500g (1lb 2oz) carrots, thinly sliced
squeeze of fresh orange juice
1 tsp maple syrup or rice syrup
salt and black pepper, to taste
1 tbsp sesame seeds, toasted, to garnish

1. Heat the oils in a large sauté pan, add the mustard seeds, and fry over a medium heat until they start to pop. Add the turmeric and ground coriander and fry for 1 minute, stirring frequently.

2. Add the carrots, orange juice, maple or rice syrup, and 2 tbsp of water, cover with a lid, and cook over a low heat for 5–10 minutes or until the carrots are tender.

3. Season to taste and scatter with toasted sesame seeds before serving.

Coriander and coconut chutney

This chutney mixture has a beautifully vibrant green colour.
It is delicious with curries and also with pies and quiches.

Serves 4

30g (1oz) grated or desiccated coconut
2 tbsp finely grated fresh ginger root
2 tsp honey or maple syrup
½ tsp salt and ½ tsp freshly ground black pepper
120ml (4fl oz) fresh lemon juice (about 1½ lemons)
2–3 large bunches fresh coriander leaves and stems, finely chopped

1. Put the coconut, ginger, honey or maple syrup, salt, and pepper into a blender and blend for 1–2 minutes. Gradually add the lemon juice and 120ml (4fl oz) filtered water and blend until the mixture forms a paste.

2. Add to the chopped coriander and mix well (do not add the coriander to the blender because the mixture becomes too liquid).

3. Leave for at least 20 minutes before serving to allow the coriander to absorb all the flavour. If the chutney appears too dry, add a few more squeezes of lemon juice – it should have more of a moist salad consistency than the jam-like texture of shop-bought chutneys. It can be kept in the refrigerator for up to 48 hours.

Raita

This is delicious served with curry; the addition of ginger helps
to stimulate digestion.

Serves 4

1 tsp ground fennel seeds
½ tsp ground ginger
500g (1lb 2oz) plain organic yogurt
2 tbsp chopped fresh coriander leaves
140g (5oz) cucumber, peeled and coarsely grated
⅓ tsp salt
¼ tsp ground black pepper

1. Dry roast the fennel seeds in a pan over medium heat for 5 minutes. Remove from the pan and grind coarsely in an electric coffee grinder.

2. In a bowl, stir together the fennel, ginger, yogurt, coriander, and cucumber. Season to taste with salt and pepper.

3. Cover and refrigerate for at least 30 minutes before serving.

Gomasio

Sprinkling gomasio on your food is a good way of reducing salt
consumption and adding healthy oils to your diet.

Makes 140g (5oz)

140g (5oz) unhulled sesame seeds
1 tsp rock salt

1. Dry roast the sesame seeds in a pan over a medium heat, stirring continually, until they give off a pleasant aroma and turn a light golden colour (about 3–5 minutes). Be careful not to let them burn.

2. Add 1 tsp salt, or to taste.

3. Coarsely grind the seeds and salt in an electric spice or coffee grinder (not one used regularly for coffee). Store in an airtight jar and shake before using. Gomasio will keep for a week to 10 days in a cool, dark cupboard or the refrigerator. It is delicious sprinkled on salads, vegetables, and soups.

Dinner

According to yoga and the science of ayurveda, the evening meal should be light and easy to digest, as our digestive capacity is not as strong at night and our metabolism slows. As a result, a heavy, late evening meal may place a burden on your liver, leading to the formation of toxins, or *ama*. Eat three hours before bedtime and avoid dairy produce and big servings of pulses; soups, pastas, and stews are good options. Try these recipes and see if you wake in the morning with more energy for the day ahead.

Stuffed butternut squash with sage

While butternut squash is not one of the most tempting squashes in appearance, its homely exterior belies its delicious taste.

Serves 4

2 butternut squash, approximately
750g (1lb 10oz) each
2 tbsp sesame oil
200g (7oz) brown rice
4 tbsp sunflower seeds, toasted
2 tsp gomasio (see p237)
large bunch fresh parsley, chopped
large bunch fresh sage, chopped
salt and freshly ground black pepper
2 tsp maple syrup
200g (7oz) feta cheese (optional)

1. Preheat the oven to 200°C (400°F/Gas 6).

2. Cut the squashes in half and place flesh-side up in a lightly oiled baking tray. Drizzle with sesame oil and bake for 45–60 minutes until tender.

3. Towards the end of the cooking time for the squashes, put the brown rice on to cook. Add 600ml (1 pint) filtered water and a pinch of salt to the rice, bring to the boil, cover, and reduce the heat to low. Cook for about 25 minutes, until all the water has been absorbed and the rice grains are soft.

4. When the squashes are cooked, remove the seeds and discard them. Spoon out the flesh, taking care not to damage the skin. Mix the flesh with the cooked rice and remaining ingredients. Spoon back into the squash and return to the oven for a further 10–15 minutes.

5. Serve with a green salad or steamed seasonal green vegetables.

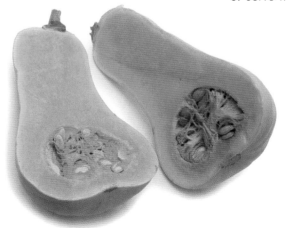

BUTTERNUT SQUASH
Sweet tasting, it is
also a source of
vitamins A and C.

Tomato, red lentil, and barley soup

The combination of lentils, root vegetables, and fragrant spices makes this thick soup a well-balanced, tasty, and filling meal.

Serves 4

1 tsp cumin seeds
1 tsp coriander seeds
1 tbsp olive oil
¼ tsp ground turmeric
2 tsp fresh ginger root, grated
1 celery stick, diced
150g (5½oz) swede, finely diced
150g (5½oz) celeriac, finely diced
1 large carrot, diced
3 large vine-ripened tomatoes, skinned and chopped
salt and freshly ground black pepper
2 sprigs rosemary
2 bay leaves
1 litre (1¾ pints) hot vegetable stock or hot, filtered water
60g (2oz) pot barley, rinsed
115g (4oz) red lentils, rinsed and soaked in water for about 30 minutes
2–3 tbsp fresh parsley, roughly chopped, to serve

1. Heat a small frying pan over medium heat, add the cumin and coriander seeds and dry fry for 1 minute or until fragrant. Tip into a mortar and pestle and grind to a powder. Heat the olive oil in a large saucepan, add the ground spices, turmeric, and ginger and fry for 1–2 minutes.

2. Add the celery, swede, celeriac, and carrots and fry, stirring frequently, for 4–5 minutes. Add the tomatoes and cook for 2–3 minutes.

3. Rinse the pot barley in lots of cold running water, add to the pot with the rosemary, bay leaves, and hot stock or water, stir well and bring to the boil. Reduce the heat to medium, and cook for 20 minutes.

4. Drain the soaked lentils and add them to the pot. Stir, bring back to the boil, then reduce the heat and simmer for 25 minutes or until the lentils are tender. Add a little more hot stock or water if the soup is too thick.

5. Remove the bay leaves and rosemary sprigs, scatter with chopped parsley, and serve hot.

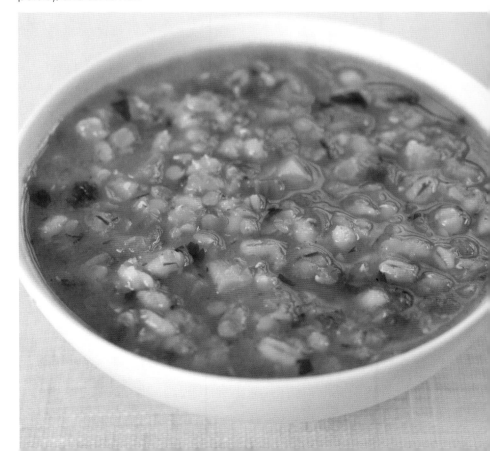

Kicharee

This simple stew is traditionally used as a healing food in a yogic diet, being a very balanced but easily digested food.

Serves 4

150g (5½ oz) yellow or green mung dhal (split mung beans)

300g (10oz) white basmati rice

2 tsp sesame oil or ghee (clarified butter)

½ tsp each of black mustard seeds, cumin seeds, ground cumin, ground coriander, and turmeric

5cm (2in) fresh root ginger, chopped

salt to taste

grated coconut, chopped fresh coriander, or a squeeze of lime, to garnish (optional)

1. It may be necessary to soak the dhal for a few hours or overnight – check the packet instructions.

2. Wash the rice and dhal together at least 3 times, until the water runs clear.

3. Heat the oil or ghee and mustard seeds in a large pan until the seeds begin to pop. Add the remaining spices and ginger and cook for 2 minutes, stirring so that the seeds do not burn.

4. Add 750ml (1¼ pints) filtered water and the rice, dhal, and salt. Bring to the boil and cook for 10 minutes.

5. Cover, reduce the heat, and simmer until the dhal and rice are soft (about 10 minutes), adding additional water if needed.

6. Garnish, if desired, with grated coconut, coriander, or a squeeze of lime.

Courgette and quinoa risotto

The courgette and cauliflower work well together in this dish, but this recipe is equally good using broccoli instead of cauliflower.

Serves 4

200g (7oz) quinoa

650ml (3½fl oz) vegetable stock or hot, filtered water

1 tsp coriander seeds

1 tsp cumin seeds

2 tsp sesame oil

1 tbsp olive oil

1 tbsp grated ginger

1 tsp turmeric

1 large courgette, chopped into bite-size pieces

150g (5½oz) cauliflower, cut into florets

2 large vine-ripened tomatoes, skinned and chopped

squeeze fresh lemon juice

salt and freshly ground black pepper

2 tbsp pine nuts

2 tbsp pumpkin seeds

2 tbsp fresh coriander or flat leaf parsley, roughly chopped, plus some whole leaves to garnish

1. Wash the quinoa thoroughly in cold water, then place the rinsed quinoa into a medium saucepan over a medium heat and fry for 1-2 minutes to toast the grains. Add the stock or hot water, stir well, and simmer over a medium heat for 15 minutes or until tender and all the stock has been absorbed. Set aside.

2. Heat a sauté pan over a medium heat, add the coriander seeds and cumin seeds, and dry fry for about 1 minute or until aromatic, stirring frequently. Tip into a mortar and pestle and grind to a powder. Heat the oils in the sauté pan, add the ground spices, ginger, and turmeric, and fry for 1-2 minutes. Add the courgette and sauté for 3-4 minutes or until just tender.

3. Meanwhile steam the cauliflower florets for 3-4 minutes or until tender.

4. While the cauliflower is cooking, heat a sauté pan over a medium heat, add the pine nuts and pumpkin seeds, and dry fry for about 1 minute, stirring frequently, until lightly toasted and fragrant.

5. Stir in the steamed cauliflower, chopped tomatoes, and lemon juice into the courgette mix, season to taste, and cook for 1-2 minutes. Stir in the pine nuts, pumpkin seeds, chopped coriander or parsley, and the cooked quinoa,

Tofu pesto

This quick and easy pesto is delicious with either wholewheat
pasta or gluten-free varieties made from quinoa, corn, or brown rice.

Serves 4

350g (12oz) silken tofu

large bunch of fresh herbs such as basil,
parsley, or mint, stalks removed

1 tbsp cold-pressed mixed seed or
olive oil

1 tbsp sesame tahini

squeeze of lemon juice, to taste

freshly ground black pepper

1. Place all the ingredients in a blender with 3 tbsp filtered water and
process until smooth and creamy – do not over-blend as this will spoil the
delicate flavour of the herbs. Adjust the consistency to taste by adding more
water if necessary.

Pumpkin, courgette, and sweet potato stew with bulghur wheat

The presence of members of the squash family and sweet potato
makes this a sweetly flavourful stew.

Serves 4

350g (12oz) pumpkin or butternut
squash

350g (12oz) sweet potatoes

350g (12oz) courgettes

1–2 tbsp ghee (clarified butter)

½ tsp each of cumin seeds, coriander
seeds, fennel seeds, and ground turmeric

1 tsp herbes de Provence

salt and freshly ground black pepper

200g (7oz) bulghur wheat

1. Peel all the vegetables and chop into bite-sized chunks.

2. Heat the ghee in a large saucepan and add the spices. Stir and cook the
spices slightly until the aroma is released.

3. Add the pumpkin or butternut squash and sweet potato and sauté for
about 5 minutes, stirring to coat with the spices.

4. Add 750ml (1¼ pints) filtered water, the herbs, and about ⅓ tsp salt and ¼
tsp pepper. Bring to the boil, turn down the heat, and simmer slowly for about
15 minutes.

5. Add the chopped courgettes, bring back to the boil, and then simmer
slowly for a further 15–25 minutes until the vegetables are cooked.

6. While the stew is cooking, prepare the bulgur wheat. Rinse thoroughly until
the water runs clear. Place 500ml (16fl oz) filtered water into a medium-sized
pan and bring to the boil. Add the bulghur wheat and a pinch of salt and
then cook on a low heat, covered, for 15 minutes.

7. When the vegetables in the stew are cooked, check the seasoning, then
serve the stew poured over the bulgur wheat.

Basic vegetable soup

Using this basic recipe, you can change the vegetables and spices according to the season and to your own tastes.

Serves 4

For the base

2 tbsp sesame oil or ghee (clarified butter)

1 tsp each ground cumin, coriander, and fennel

1 tsp mixed herbs or turmeric, depending on the desired flavour

For the vegetables

300g (10oz) in-season vegetables, chopped into small pieces

100g (3½oz) potato or other thickener if needed, peeled and chopped into small pieces

For the liquid

1 litre (1¾ pints) filtered water or cooking vegetable liquid, or a mixture of water and soya milk

salt and freshly ground black pepper

For the garnish

Choose from chopped fresh herbs, crème fraîche, gomasio (see p237) flaked nori, or toasted seaweed

1. Heat the oil or ghee gently in a large saucepan, then add the spices and stir until the aromas are released.

2. Add the vegetables and stir to coat them in the oil and spices. Sauté gently for 3–5 minutes until they are softened.

3. Add three-quarters of the liquid, saving the rest for thinning down if necessary, and season with salt and pepper. Bring to the boil, then simmer gently for about 20 minutes until all the vegetables are tender.

4. Liquidize if a smooth soup is desired and then return to the pan. Add the rest of the liquid if needed to reach the desired consistency and adjust seasoning to taste.

5. Serve garnished with your choice of chopped fresh herbs, crème fraîche, gomasio, nori, or toasted seaweed.

Creamy sweet potato and carrot soup

Use desiccated coconut to make your own coconut milk, and experiment with exotic flavours in this fragrant soup.

Serves 4

150g (5½oz) desiccated coconut

2 tsp grated fresh root ginger

500g (1lb 2oz) sweet potatoes, finely chopped

500g (1lb 2oz) carrots, finely chopped

1 litre (1¾ pints) vegetable stock

freshly ground black pepper

fresh coriander leaves, to garnish

1. The coconut milk can be made in advance and stored for 24 hours in the refrigerator, or you can make it as you prepare the soup. Place the desiccated coconut in a bowl and pour 500ml (16fl oz) boiling filtered water over it. Stir to combine and leave to soak for 10 minutes, then whizz in a blender on high for 1 minute. Leave for a further 10 minutes and then pass through a sieve into a bowl, using the back of a spoon to squeeze out all the excess moisture. Discard the coconut remaining in the sieve.

2. Place the ginger, sweet potatoes, and carrots in a medium-sized pan and add the vegetable stock. Bring to the boil, reduce the heat, and simmer for about 15 minutes until the vegetables are soft.

3. Purée the soup in a blender with the coconut milk and black pepper. Serve garnished with fresh coriander.

Barley risotto

One of the best sources of soluble and insoluble fibre, barley makes this risotto especially healthy.

Serves 4

1 tbsp olive oil or ghee (clarified butter)

3cm (1¼ in) fresh ginger root

200g (7oz) pot barley

600 ml (1 pint) hot vegetable stock or filtered water

140g (5oz) fresh or frozen peas

85g (3oz) asparagus, bottoms trimmed and stalk finely chopped, leaving 2–3cm (¾ –1¼ in) stem below the tips (set aside ⅔ of the asparagus tips)

small handful of mint leaves, shredded

pinch of rock salt and freshly ground black pepper

vegetarian Parmesan cheese, grated

reserved asparagus tips, blanched in boiling water for 1 minute

mint leaves, to garnish

1. Place the olive oil or ghee in a large saucepan over a moderate heat. When the oil is hot, add the ginger and pot barley to the pan and cook, stirring regularly, for 2–3 minutes.

2. Gradually stir in half the hot stock. Bring the stock to a steady simmer and leave to cook for 15 minutes, stirring regularly, until almost all the stock has been absorbed. Add the rest of the stock to the barley and repeat the process for a further 15–20 minutes, at which time the barley should be tender with a little bite to it and the stock should be mainly absorbed. If the barley is still firm, add a little more stock or water and allow it to cook for a further 5–10 minutes.

3. Stir in the peas and chopped asparagus and cook them with the barley for 5 minutes until they are tender.

4. Remove the risotto from the heat and stir in the mint and seasoning until well distributed.

5. To serve, divide the risotto between 4 serving bowls and place the blanched asparagus tips in the centre of each bowl. Scatter the grated Parmesan over the top and sprinkle with mint leaves to garnish.

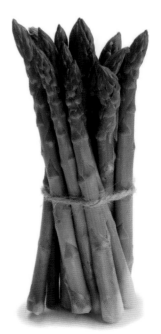

ASPARAGUS
This delicately flavoured vegetable is high in folate and vitamins A and C.

Breads

Wholegrain breads are a good source of fibre, B vitamins, and protein. If you are reluctant to eat wheat or yeast, you will be able to find alternative grains in health food shops – and the recipes given here are all yeast-free.

Pumpkin soda bread

This bread is delicious served warm, sliced and spread with butter. If you cannot find spelt flour, use wholemeal flour instead.

Makes 1 large loaf

175g (6oz) self-raising flour
150g (5½oz) spelt flour
150g (5½oz) wholemeal flour
1 tsp bicarbonate of soda
1 tsp salt
1 tsp honey
50g (1¾oz) pumpkin or butternut squash, grated
3 tbsp of mixed seeds, made up of 1 tbsp pumpkin seeds, toasted, and 2 tbsp sesame or sunflower seeds, toasted
400ml (14fl oz) buttermilk or plain natural yogurt

1. Preheat the oven to 200°C (400°F/Gas 6). In a large bowl, sift together the flours and bicarbonate of soda, then stir in the salt, honey, grated pumpkin, and 1 tablespoon of the mixed seeds.

2. Make a well in the middle of the dry mix and stir in 375ml (13fl oz) of the buttermilk or natural yogurt and stir with a wooden spoon to form a loose dough. Tip onto a lightly floured surface and gently knead into a ball.

3. Lightly score a cross on the top of the bread, then brush with the rest of the buttermilk and scatter over the remaining seeds. Place on a greased baking sheet and bake for 30–35 minutes or until when you tap the underside of the loaf it produces a hollow sound. Turn out onto a wire rack, wrap in a clean tea-towel, and leave to cool slightly before serving.

Alex's buckwheat pitta breads

These gluten-free pitta breads are quick to make and go well with soups and main meals, or with jam or nut butters for breakfast.

Makes 8

150g (5½oz) buckwheat flour
pinch of salt
¼ tsp finely ground black pepper
pinch of ground turmeric (optional)
fresh basil or sage, chopped (optional)

1. Place the flour, salt, pepper, and turmeric in a bowl and gradually add about 250ml (8fl oz) filtered water, beating with a hand whisk to remove any lumps and to ensure there is plenty of air in the batter. The mixture should have a consistency slightly thicker than a pancake batter. Stir in the herbs, if using. Cover and refrigerate for a few hours or overnight.

2. Heat a non-stick pan on a medium heat – if it is too hot, the batter surface will cook too quickly and the grain inside will remain uncooked. Add 1 tbsp batter. When the top is dry, flip over. Continue cooking until the pitta is solid enough to be put into a toaster – a few minutes at most.

3. Pop the pitta into the toaster for a minute – it will puff up with air. Keep warm on a wire rack while you cook the rest. Eat within 30 minutes.

Chapati

These Indian flatbreads are a great accompaniment to main meals, but can be served at any time of day.

Makes 10

150g (5½ oz) wholewheat or special chapati flour

½ tsp salt

1 tsp ghee (clarified butter) or 2 tsp sunflower oil

1. In a deep bowl, mix the flour, salt, and ghee or oil, using your hands.

2. Gradually add 75ml (2½fl oz) filtered water, mixing to form a slightly sticky dough. Knead for 5–10 minutes. Cover the bowl with a damp cloth and leave to rest in the refrigerator overnight or for at least 2 hours.

3. Divide the dough into 10 and knead into balls between your hands. Cover with flour before rolling out into thin discs about 12cm (5in) in diameter. Cook one at a time in a hot iron pan over medium heat. Turn after 30 seconds (or when you see small bubbles) and cook for another 30 seconds.

4. If using a gas stove, hold the chapati with tongs and wave each one over an open flame for a few seconds until it puffs up. On an electric stove, roll a clean tea-towel into a ball and press it hard into the chapati in the pan.

5. To keep the chapatis warm for a few hours, wrap in a tea-towel and then place in a plastic bag in a crockery dish. Spread with ghee to serve.

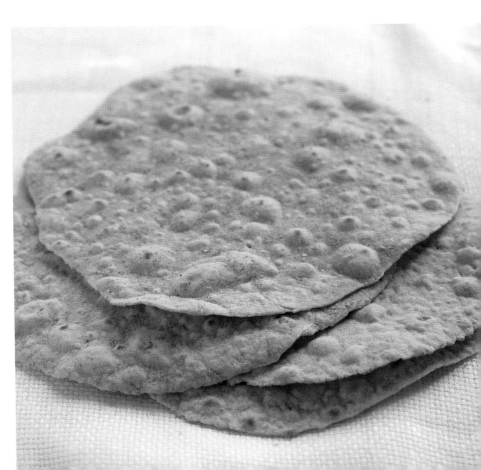

Sweet treats and desserts

Sweets should be used as occasional treats, and not as staple foods. In that context, especially when served as part of a celebration or with friends and family, they should be eaten with joy, love, and an easy conscience! Using non-refined sweeteners such as cinnamon, honey, maple syrup, and coconut rather than sugar, these dessert recipes are tasty, satisfying, and good for the soul.

Saffron rice

Rice pudding is sometimes unfairly regarded as a worthy but rather dull dish. This recipe is a spicy version.

Serves 4

150g (5½oz) white basmati rice, uncooked

750ml (1¼ pints) organic cow's or goat's milk

pinch of saffron threads

seeds of 2 cardamom pods

½ tsp ground cloves

3 tbsp maple syrup or brown rice syrup

2 tbsp shredded coconut

grated zest of 1 lemon, to garnish

1. Wash the rice the until water runs clear.

2. Combine the rice, milk, saffron, cardamom seeds, and ground cloves in a large pan. Bring to the boil, then reduce the heat and simmer over a low heat for 30 minutes.

3. To toast the coconut, dry fry in a pan over medium heat, stirring frequently, until golden.

4. Once cooked, stir in the syrup to taste and serve topped with the coconut and lemon zest. The pudding may be served hot or cold.

Chocolate and silken tofu mousse

This dessert seems to be too good to be true – deliciously creamy, yet low in fat and sugar and high in calcium and phytoestrogens.

Serves 4

150g (5½oz) bar organic dark chocolate (you can use plain or flavoured versions, such as chocolate with orange)

350g (12oz) pack silken tofu

grated zest of 1 orange

grated chocolate or chopped nuts, to garnish

1. Break the chocolate into squares and place in a small bowl with 3 tsp filtered water. Place this bowl over a pan of simmering water and gradually stir until the chocolate has melted.

2. Put the silken tofu into a blender, add the melted chocolate and orange zest, and blend until all the chocolate is mixed in.

3. Pour the mixture into individual ramekins and place in the refrigerator for 2–6 hours to set.

4. Before serving, sprinkle with grated chocolate or some chopped nuts.

Fruit crumble

Here apples and blackberries are used, but you can include any
of your favourite fruits as the base.

Serves 4

For the filling

4 large cooking apples, peeled, cored,
and diced

225g (8oz) blackberries

4 tbsp raisins (optional)

1 tsp ground cinnamon

zest of ½ lemon, grated

For the topping

100g (3½oz) rolled oats

75g (2½oz) wholewheat flour

50g (1¾oz) organic butter

100ml (3½fl oz) maple syrup

organic single cream (optional)

1. Preheat the oven to 190°C (375°F/Gas 5). Butter a 20cm (8 inch) square,
ovenproof dish.

2. Mix all the filling ingredients together and place in the baking dish.

3. To make the topping, combine the oats and flour. Heat the butter and
maple syrup until the butter has melted. Stir this mixture into the oats and mix
well. Spoon the topping over the filling.

4. Place in the oven and bake for about 50 minutes – the filling should be
soft but not too runny. Serve with single cream, if desired.

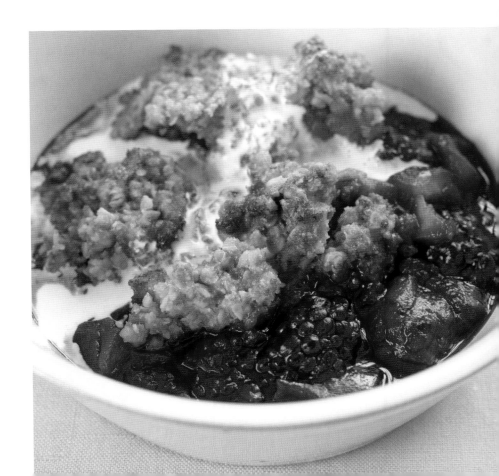

Snacks and beverages

Snacks are not recommended in yoga, as eating between meals is thought to reduce digestive capacity and place an unnecessary burden on the body. However, with the hectic schedules that many of us follow today, healthy snacks may be necessary from time to time. To avoid commercial products that are high in sugar, salt, and fat, try these easily prepared alternatives or snack on fruit, nuts, and seeds.

Dry-roasted chickpeas with spice

Chickpeas are popular for snacks as they are very sustaining. Here they are warmly spiced with coriander.

Makes 350g (12oz)

200g (7oz) dried chickpeas, soaked overnight in 1 litre (1¾ pints) filtered water

1 tsp ground coriander

½ tsp salt

vegetable oil, for greasing

1. Drain the water from the soaked chickpeas and rinse them well. Add them to a pan with 750ml (1¼ pints) water and bring to the boil. Simmer, covered, for 1½ hours and then drain.

2. Preheat the oven to 160°C (325°F/Gas 3).

3. Mix the cooked chickpeas with the coriander and salt and spread on a lightly oiled baking tray.

4. Place in the oven for 45 minutes or until the chickpeas are crisp on the outside and slightly tender inside.

Avocado and tofu dip

If you use silken tofu, you may not need quite as much soya milk in this recipe to get the desired creaminess.

Serves 4

300g (10oz) silken or ordinary tofu

2 small ripe avocados

6 tbsp freshly chopped parsley

2 tsp tamari or soy sauce

freshly ground black pepper (to taste)

150–200ml (5–7fl oz) soya milk

selection of raw vegetables, for dipping

1. Process all the ingredients (apart from the vegetables for dipping) in a blender until smooth, adding as much soya milk as you need to achieve the desired consistency.

2. Dip the vegetables in to serve. Carrot sticks go very well with the flavours of this dip, but you can use any fresh vegetables you have to hand.

Miso and hazelnut spread

This spread is delicious on crackers or toast for breakfast or as a
light snack. It also makes a good sandwich filling with watercress.

Serves 4

4 tbsp hazelnuts
1 tbsp light fresh miso

1. Roast the hazelnuts in a hot pan over a high heat, until slightly brown, stirring continuously to stop them burning.

2. Put them in a blender with the miso and 3 tbsp filtered water, and blend until smooth.

Chai

This spicy drink with zesty, complex flavours is a great substitute
when you are trying to give up coffee.

Serves 4

2 tsp fresh root ginger, finely sliced
2 tsp whole fennel seeds
¼ tsp black peppercorns
1 fresh bay leaf
15 cardamom pods
6 whole cloves
1 cinnamon stick
1 tsp black tea leaves
8 fl oz (250 ml) almond milk
4 tsp honey

1. In a saucepan, combine 750ml (24fl oz) cold, filtered water with the ginger, fennel seeds, black peppercorns, bay leaf, cardamom pods, cloves, and cinnamon stick. Bring to the boil, then cover, reduce the heat and simmer for 5 minutes. Take the pan off the heat, add the tea, and let it steep for 5-10 minutes.

2. Strain the tea through a sieve into a large jug, add the almond milk and honey, and serve immediately.

Almond milk

A great energizer and source of calcium, and with a light, nutty
taste, almond milk is refreshing served chilled on a hot day.

Serves 4

140g (5oz) organic almonds
1 tsp ground cardamom
4 tsp honey

1. First you will need to remove the skins from the almonds by blanching them. To do this, put the almonds in a bowl and pour over boiling water to cover. Leave them to soak for about 4-5 minutes, then drain off the water. The moistened skins should now slip off easily by squeezing the almonds between your thumb and fingers. Discard the skins.

2. Put the almonds, 500ml (16fl oz) filtered water, cardamom, and honey into a blender and whizz on high speed until the mix reaches a creamy consistency.

3. Strain the liquid from the pulp through a sieve lined with cheesecloth. The almond milk will keep refrigerated for up to 2-3 days.

Resources

International Sivananda Yoga
Vedanta Centres and Ashrams
Founder: Swami Vishnudevananda

www.sivananda.org

Ashrams

HEADQUARTERS: CANADA

Sivananda Ashram Yoga Camp
673, 8th Avenue Val Morin
Quebec J0T 2R0,
Canada
Tel: +1.819.322.3226
e-mail: HQ@sivananda.org

AUSTRIA

Sivananda Yoga Retreat House
Bichlach 40
A- 6370 Reith bei Kitzbühel
Tyrol
Austria
Tel: +435.356.674.04
e-mail: tyrol@sivananda.net

BAHAMAS

Sivananda Ashram Yoga Retreat
P.O. Box N7550 Paradise Island
Nassau, Bahamas
Tel: +1.242.363.2902
e-mail: Nassau@sivananda.org

FRANCE

Château du Yoga Sivananda
26 Impasse du Bignon
45170 Neuville aux bois
France
Tel: +33.238.918.882
e-mail: orleans@sivananda.net

INDIA

Sivananda Yoga Vedanta
Meenakshi Ashram
Near Pavanna Vilakku Junction,
New Natham Road
Saramthangi Village
Madurai Dist. 625 503
Tamil Nadu, South India
Tel: +91.944.2190.661
e-mail: madurai@sivananda.org

Sivananda Kutir
(Near Siror Bridge)
P.O. Netala, Uttar Kashi Dt,
Uttaranchal, Himalayas, 249 193,
North India
Tel: +91.137.4.22.4159
or +91.9411.330.495
e-mail: Himalayas@sivananda.org

Sivananda Yoga Vedanta
Dhanwantari Ashram
P.O. Neyyar Dam
Thiruvananthapuram Dt.
Kerala, 695 572, India
Tel: +91.471.227.3093/2703
e-mail: YogaIndia@sivananda.org

UNITED STATES

Sivananda Ashram Yoga Ranch
P.O. Box 195, Budd Road
Woodbourne, NY 12788, USA
Tel: +1.845.436.6492
e-mail: YogaRanch@sivananda.org

Sivananda Ashram Yoga Farm
14651 Ballantree Lane
Grass Valley, CA 95949, USA
Tel: +1.530.272.9322
e-mail: yogafarm@sivananda.org

Centres

ARGENTINA

Centro Internaciónal de Yoga Sivananda
Sánchez de Bustamante 2372 -
(C.P. 1425)
Capital Federal - Buenos Aires -
Argentina
Tel: +54.114.804. 7813
e-mail: BuenosAires@sivananda.org

AUSTRIA

Sivananda Yoga Vedanta Zentrum
Prinz Eugen Strasse 18
A -1040 Vienna, Austria
Tel:: +43.158.63453
e-mail: vienna@sivananda.net

CANADA

Sivananda Yoga Vedanta Centre
5178 St Lawrence Blvd
Montreal
Quebec H2T 1R8, Canada
Tel: +1.514.279.3545
e-mail: Montreal@sivananda.org

Sivananda Yoga Vedanta Centre
77 Harbord Street
Toronto
Ontario M5S 1G4, Canada
Tel: +1.416.966.9642
e-mail: Toronto@sivananda.org

FRANCE

Centre Sivananda de Yoga Vedanta
140 rue du Faubourg Saint-Martin
F-75010 Paris
France
Tel: +33.140.267.749
e-mail: Paris@sivananda.net

GERMANY

Sivananda Yoga Vedanta Zentrum
Steinheilstrasse 1
D-80333 Munich, Germany
Tel: +49.897.009.6690
e-mail: Munich@sivananda.net

Sivananda Yoga Vedanta Zentrum
Schmiljanstrasse 24
D-12161 Berlin, Germany
Tel: +49.308.599.9798
e-mail: Berlin@sivananda.net

INDIA

Sivananda Yoga Vedanta Nataraja Centre
A-41 Kailash Colony
New Delhi 110 048, India
Tel: +91.112.924.0869
or +91.112.923.0962
e-mail: Delhi@sivananda.org

Sivananda Yoga Vedanta Dwarka Centre
PSP Pocket, Swami Sivananda Marg,
Sector - 6 (Behind DAV school)
Dwarka, New Delhi 110075, India
Tel: +91.116.456.8526
Or +91.114.556.6016
e-mail: Dwarka@sivananda.org

Sivananda Yoga Vedanta Centre
TC37/1927 (5), Airport Road
West Fort,
Thiruvananthapuram Kerala, India
Tel +91.047.124.50942
+91.9497.008.432
e-mail: trivandrum@sivananda.org

Sivananda Yoga Vedanta Centre
3/655 Kaveri Nagar, Kuppam Road,
Kottivakkam
Chennai 600 041, Tamil Nadu, India
Tel: +91.442.451.1626
or +91.442.451.2546
e-mail: Chennai@sivananda.org

Sivananda Yoga Vedanta Centre
Plot # 101 (Old No 23)
Dr Sathar Road
Anna Nagar, Madurai 625 020
Tamil Nadu, India
Tel: +91.452.252.1170
e-mail: maduraicentre@sivananda.org

ISRAEL

Sivananda Yoga Vedanta Centre
6 Lateris St
Tel Aviv 64166
Israel
Tel: +972.3.691.6793
e-mail: TelAviv@sivananda.org

ITALY

Centro Yoga Vedanta Sivananda Roma
via Oreste Tommasini, 7
00162 Rome
Italy
tel: +39.064.549.6529
e-mail: roma@sivananda.org

Centro Yoga Vedanta Sivananda Milano
Milan, Italy
Phone: +39.334.760.5376
e-mail: Milan@sivananda.org

LITHUANIA

Šivananda jogos vedantos centras
Vivulskio g. 41
03114 Vilnius
Lithuania
e-mail: vilnius@sivananda.net

SPAIN

Centro de Yoga Sivananda Vedanta
Calle Eraso 4
E-28028 Madrid
Spain
Tel: +34.913.615.150
e-mail: Madrid@sivananda.net

SWITZERLAND

Centre Sivananda de Yoga Vedanta
1 Rue des Minoteries
CH-1205 Geneva, Switzerland
Tel: +41.223.280.3
28
e-mail: Geneva@sivananda.net

UNITED KINGDOM

Sivananda Yoga Vedanta Centre
51 Felsham Road
London SW15 1AZ
Tel: +44.208.780.0160
e-mail: London@sivananda.net

UNITED STATES

Sivananda Yoga Vedanta Center
1246 West Bryn Mawr Avenue
Chicago, IL 60660, USA
Tel: +1.773.878.7771
e-mail: Chicago@sivananda.org

Sivananda Yoga Vedanta Center
243 West 24th Street
New York, NY 10011, USA
Tel: +1.212.255.4560
e-mail: NewYork@sivananda.org

Sivananda Yoga Vedanta Center
1200 Arguello Blvd
San Francisco, CA 94122, USA
Tel: +1.415.681.2731
e-mail: SanFrancisco@sivananda.org

Sivananda Yoga Vedanta Center
13325 Beach Avenue
Marina del Rey, CA 90292, USA
Tel: +1.310.822.9642
e-mail: LosAngeles@sivananda.org

URUGUAY

Asociación de Yoga Sivananda
Acevedo Díaz 1523
11200 Montevideo, Uruguay
Tel: +598.240.109.29/401.6685
e-mail: Montevideo@sivananda.org

Index

A

Abdominal Breathing 180
acid-alkaline balance 215
adrenaline 34, 205
affirmations 206–7
agonist muscles 21
air, element 18
almond milk 249
Alternate Nostril Breathing 182–3
antagonist muscles 21
apples: fruit crumble 247
asanas 10, 11, 12, 14, 44–5, 46–7
astral energy channels 178
aura 178
autonomic nervous system 34–5
autosuggestion, relaxation 38
avocado and tofu dip 248

B

bananas: buckwheat banana
    pancakes 225
  breakfast muffins 223
barley: barley risotto 243
  tomato, red lentil, and barley
    soup 239
beans, cooking techniques 219
Bhakti yoga 10
blackberries: fruit crumble 247
blueberries: buckwheat banana
    pancakes 225
Boat 36, 124
Boat with Interlock 125
Bound Half Lotus Forward Bend 105
Bow 29, 134–9
breads 244–5
breakfast 220–21, 222–5
breakfast muffins 223
breathing 32–3, 176–85

Abdominal Breathing 180
Alternate Nostril Breathing 182–3
breath-control 15, 33
during meditation 203
Full Yogic Breath 181
hyperventilation 184
involuntary breathing 32
Kapala Bhati 184–5
stress management 205
voluntary breath-control 33
yogic breathing 12, 176–85
Bridge 86–9
buckwheat: Alex's buckwheat pitta
    breads 244
  buckwheat banana pancakes
    225
bulghur wheat, pumpkin, courgette,
    and sweet potato stew with 241
burgers, millet 231
Butterfly 102
butternut squash with sage 238

C

cabbage: coleslaw 234
calcium 210, 215
Californian wrap 233
Camel 20–21, 128
candles, meditation 202
carbohydrates 214
cardiovascular system 40
carrots: carrot and raisin salad 234
  creamy sweet potato and carrot
    soup 242
  sweet sesame carrots 236
chai 249
chakras 179, 204
chapati 245
cheese: pea and quinoa salad 227
  roasted Tuscan wraps 233

stuffed butternut squash with
    sage 238
chickpeas: vegetable coconut curry
    229
  dry-roasted chickpeas with
    spice 248
  roasted vegetables and chickpeas
    226
Child's Pose 191
Chin Mudra 204
chocolate and silken tofu
    mousse 246
chutney, coriander and coconut 237
clothing 45
Cobra 29, 116–21
coconut: coriander and coconut
    chutney 237
  vegetable coconut curry 229
coleslaw, walnut 234
concentration 200–201, 204
condiments 237
connective tissue 26–7
contractions, muscles 21–5, 38
coriander and coconut chutney 237
Corpse Pose 38, 46, 188, 192–3
cosmic consciousness 198
counterposes 45
courgette: courgette and quinoa
    risotto 240
  courgette, pumpkin, and sweet
    potato stew 241
couscous, roasted vegetables, and
    chickpeas with 226
Crescent Moon 132–3
Crescent Splits 112–13
cross-legged pose 203
Crow 150–53
cucumber: raita 237

D

dairy produce 211, 214
Dancing Lord Siva 160–61
dhal, sweet cinnamon 228
Diagonal Shooting Bow 110
Diamond 129
diaphragm, Abdominal
  Breathing 180
diet 13, 15, 208–49
  common concerns 214–15
  cooking techniques 218–19
  eating with awareness 212–13
  menus 220–21
  recipes 222–49
  transition to yogic diet 216–17
  vegetarianism 210–21
digestive system 40
dinner 220–21, 238–43
dip, avocado and tofu 248
disease, causes of 18
dizziness 184
Dolphin 62–3
Double Leg Lifts 30, 60–1
dressings 235
dried fruit: breakfast muffins 223
  dried fruit compôte 224
  morning energy shake 225
drinks 249

E

Eagle 159
earth, element 18
eccentric contraction, muscles 24–5
ego 198
elements 18
emotions 18, 198, 206
endocrine system 18, 37, 40
energy: negative thoughts 206
  prana 178
ether, element 18
eye exercises 48

F

fascia 26–7
fear 206
"fight or flight" response 34, 205
fire, element 18
Fish 29, 92–5, 115
five elements 18
flatbreads, Indian 245
food see diet
Forward Bend 96–9
  Bound Half Lotus Forward
  Bend 105
  correcting lordosis 30
  Forward Bend Lotus Headstand 71
  Half Lotus Forward Bend 103
  relaxing in 189
  Single Leg Forward Bend 102
  Standing Forward Bend 162–3
  Straight Arm Forward Bend 105
fruit 211
fruit crumble 247
Full Yogic Breath 181

G

gomasio 237
grains, cooking techniques 218
granola, crispy 224
gunas 212–13

H

Half Lotus 203
Half Lotus Tree 159
Half Spinal Twist 144–9
hands, mudras 182, 183, 204
Handstand 74–5
happiness 206
Hatha yoga 10, 11
Hatha Yoga Pradipika 14–15
Headstand 19, 62–71
healing 18–19
health benefits, vegetarianism 210
heart, benefits of yoga 19
history of Sivananda yoga 8–9

homeostasis 18, 34, 198
hormones 34, 37
hyperventilation 184

I

ida nadi 178, 179
immune system 198, 205
incense 202
Inclined Plane 100–101
Indian flatbreads 245
inverted poses, benefits of 19
involuntary breathing 32
isometric contraction, muscles 22
isotonic contraction, muscles 23

J

Jnana yoga 10
joints 20–27

K

Kapala Bhati 184–5
karma, law of 206–7
Karma yoga 10
kicharee 240
King Cobra 120–21
kyphosis 29

L

lacto-vegetarian diet 210–21
Lateral Bend with Twist 107
law of karma 206–7
Leg Lifts 58–61, 106–7
Leg Stretch 36
legumes, cooking techniques 219
lemon and olive oil dressing 235
lentils: tomato, red lentil, and barley
  soup 239
  sweet cinnamon dhal 228
  vegetarian shepherd's pie 228
Locust 122–7
lordosis 30
Lotus 114–15, 203
  Bound Half Lotus Forward Bend 105

Half Lotus 203
Half Lotus Bridge 89
Half Lotus Forward Bend 103
Half Lotus Tree 159
Locust in Lotus 127
Lotus Balance 115
Lotus Fish 95
Lotus Headstand 70–71
Lotus Peacock 157
lunch 220–21, 226–33
lungs 32–3, 178, 184
Lying Fish 115

M

meat 210
meditation 13, 196–207
  benefits of 198–9
  concentration 200–201
  law of karma 206–7
  practising 202–4
  stress management 205
Mediterranean spinach 236
mental meditation 198, 204
mental relaxation 193, 195
menus 220–21
Middle Eastern wrap 233
milk: morning energy shake 225
millet: millet burgers 231
  spiced millet porridge 224
mind: concentration 200–201
  meditation 204
  relaxation 195
miso and hazlenut spread p249
mudras 182, 204
muesli, home-made 222
muffins, breakfast 223
mung beans: kicharee 240
muscles 20–27, 40
  balancing nervous system 36
  contractions 21–5, 38
  posture 28–31
  proper exercise 44
  relaxation 38–9

N

nadis 178, 179
neck exercise 49
negative thoughts 206
nervous system 18, 34–6, 40, 198, 205
noodles with stir-fry vegetables and tofu 231
noradrenaline 34, 205
nostrils, Alternate Nostril Breathing 182–3
nuts 211

O

oats: crispy granola 224
  spiced oat porridge 224
oils 219
One Foot to Head 108–9

P

pancakes, buckwheat 225
parasympathetic nervous system 34–5, 198, 205
parsley and nut or seed dressing 235
Patanjali 11
pea and quinoa salad 227
Peacock 154–7
pesto, tofu 241
physical meditation 202–3
physical relaxation 192–3, 194–5
Pigeon 130–31
Pigeon Splits 113
pilaf, asparagus quinoa 240
pingala nadi 178
pitta breads 244
plant foods 210
Plough 80–85
porridge, spiced oat or millet 224
positive thinking 13, 18, 206–7
posture 28–31
potatoes: vegetarian shepherd's pie 228
prana 178
pranayama (yogic breathing)

11, 12, 176–85
proper exercise 44–5
pulses 211
pumpkin: pumpkin, courgette, and sweet potato stew 241
  pumpkin soda bread 244

Q

quinoa: courgette and quinoa risotto 240
  pea and quinoa salad 227
  vanilla quinoa cereal 222

R

raisins: carrot and raisin salad 234
  crispy granola 224
raita 237
Raja yoga 10, 11
Rajasic foods 212–13, 215
recipes 222–49
relaxation 13, 38–9, 44, 46, 186–95
  balancing nervous system 36
  complete yogic relaxation 192–3, 194–5
  eyes 48
  final relaxation 192–93
  relaxing on your front 190
  stress management 205
respiratory system 32–3, 178–9
rice: kicharee 240
  saffron rice 246
  stuffed butternut squash with sage 238
  tofu kebabs with saffron rice 230
risotto, barley 243
Rocking Bow 136

S

saffron rice 246
salads: carrot and raisin salad 234
  pea and quinoa salad 227
  walnut coleslaw 234
samadhi (cosmic consciousness) 11, 198

Sattvic foods 212–13, 215
scoliosis 31
Scorpion 72–3
Scorpion Handstand 75
Seated One Leg Raise 106
Seated Two Leg Raise 107
seeds 211
    crispy granola 224
sequences 170–75
sesame seeds: gomasio 237
shepherd's pie, vegetarian 228
Shooting Bow 110–11
Shoulderstand 23, 37, 76–9
Shoulderstand cycle 90–91
Shoulderstand to Bridge 87
Side Crow 153
Single Leg Forward Bend 102
Single Leg Lifts 58–9
Single Nostril Breathing 182
sitting positions 203, 205
Sivananda, Swami 8
snacks 220–21, 248–9
soba noodles with stir-fry vegetables
    and tofu 231
soda bread, pumpkin 244
soups: basic vegetable soup 242
    creamy sweet potato and carrot
        soup 242
    tomato, red lentil, and barley soup
        239
space, element 18
spinach, Mediterranean 236
Spinal Twist 31, 144–9, 167
spine: kyphosis 29
    lordosis 30
    scoliosis 31
spiritual benefits, meditation 199
spiritual relaxation 193, 195
Splits 112–13
squash: stuffed butternut squash
    with sage 238
standing balances 158–61
Standing Forward Bend 26–7, 30,
    162–3

Straight Arm Forward Bend 105
Straight Leg Shooting Bow 111
stress 34, 205
stretches 36, 44
Sun Salutation 36, 50–7
sushumna nadi 178, 179
Swatmarama Yogi 14
sweet potatoes: creamy sweet
        potato and carrot soup 242
    pumpkin, courgette, and sweet
        potato stew 241
sympathetic nervous system 34–5

T
tahini dressing 235
Tamasic foods 212–13, 215
tea: chai 249
tempeh wrap 233
thoughts, law of karma 206–7
tofu: avocado and tofu dip 248
    chocolate and silken tofu
        mousse 246
    scrambled tofu and
        vegetables 225
    soba noodles with stir-fry
        vegetables and tofu 231
    tofu kebabs with saffron rice 230
    tofu pesto 241
Tortoise 106
Tree 158
    Half Lotus Tree 159
Triangle 164–9
    benefits of 40–41
    correcting scoliosis 31
    Head to Toe 169
    muscles 20–1, 22–3, 24–5
    Simple Hip Twist 166
    Triangle with Bent Knee 168
    Triangle with Spinal Twist 167
Tuscan wraps, roasted 233
Twisted Lotus Headstand 71

V
vanilla quinoa cereal 222
variations, asanas 45
vegetable coconut curry 229
vegetables 211, 236
    basic vegetable soup 242
    tomato, red lentil, and barley soup
        239
    roasted Tuscan wraps 233
    roasted vegetables and chickpeas
        with couscous 226
    scrambled tofu and
        vegetables 225
    soba noodles with stir-fry
        vegetables and tofu 231
    vegetable coconut curry 229
vegetarian shepherd's pie 228
vegetarianism 210–21
Vishnu Mudra 182
Vishnudevananda, Swami 8–9, 12
visualization 205, 207

W
water, element 18
well-being, yogic path to 12–13
Wheel 140–43
wholegrains 211
work, stress management 205

Y
yam pie with a crunchy nutty
    crust 232
yogic relaxation 194–5
yogurt: morning energy shake 225
    raita 237

Acknowledgments

AUTHOR'S ACKNOWLEDGMENTS

Swami Sivadasananda would like to thank Swami Kailasananda and Swami Durgananda for their help and advice; Prema, Satyadev, and Liese for their skill and enthusiasm in demonstrating the yoga techniques; Anne Razvi for the Proper Diet chapter; Hilary Mandleberg for the skilful editing work; and the very dedicated and enthusiastic team at DK.

To find out more about the Sivananda Yoga Vedanta Centres go to: www.sivananda.org or contact Swami Sivadasananda, e-mail: sws@sivananda.net

PUBLISHER'S ACKNOWLEDGMENTS

Dorling Kindersley would like to thank John Freeman for all the model photography; models Prema (Karina Andrea Arenas Bonansea), Satyadev (Steeve Petteau), and Liese Grillmayer; Rachel Jones for hair and makeup; Kevin Boak of Kevin Boak Studio; the Sivananda Yoga Vedanta centre, London, for the loan of props and mats; William Reavell for food photography: Cara Hobday for food styling; designers Nicky Collings, Mandy Earey, Anne Fisher, Ruth Hope, Helen McTeer; Danaya Bunnag for design assistance; Anna Burges-Lumsden for recipe testing; Susannah Marriott for additional editorial help; Annelise Evans for proofreading; Hilary Bird for the index; Peter Bull Arts Studio for the anatomical artworks.

Thanks to Anne Razvi for the Proper Diet chapter. Anne is an Ayurvedic therapist and clinical nutritionist, with practices in the UK and Spain. For more details about Anne Razvi and how to contact her, visit www.physicalnutrition.net

PICTURE CREDITS

p9 Sivananda Yoga Vendata Centre
p200 (second left) Dorling Kindersley (c) Angus Beare
All other images © Dorling Kindersley
For further information see www.dkimages.com